The
Way *of* Play

The
Way
of
Play

Using Little Moments
of Big Connection to Raise
Calm and Confident Kids

**Tina Payne Bryson, PhD,
and Georgie Wisen-Vincent, LMFT**

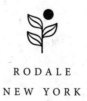

RODALE
NEW YORK

Published in the United States by Rodale Books, an imprint of
Random House, a division of Penguin Random House LLC, New York.

RODALE and the Plant colophon are registered trademarks of
Penguin Random House LLC.

LIBRARY OF CONGRESS CATALOGING-IN-PUBLICATION DATA
Names: Bryson, Tina Payne, author. | Wisen-Vincent, Georgie, author.
Title: The way of play / Tina Payne Bryson, PhD and
Georgie Wisen-Vincent, LMFT
Description: New York, NY: Rodale, 2025 | Includes index.
Identifiers: LCCN 2024015336 (print) | LCCN 2024015337 (ebook) |
ISBN 9780593796283 (hardcover) | ISBN 9780593796290 (ebook)
Subjects: LCSH: Play—Psychological aspects. | Child psychology.
Classification: LCC BF717 .B79 2024 (print) | LCC BF717 (ebook) |
DDC 155.4/18—dc23/eng/20240515
LC record available at https://lccn.loc.gov/2024015336
LC ebook record available at https://lccn.loc.gov/2024015337

Printed in the United States of America on acid-free paper

RodaleBooks.com | RandomHouseBooks.com

2 4 6 8 9 7 5 3 1

First Edition

Book design by Diane Hobbing

To Justin and Jack, you'll always be my favorite people
to play with in the whole world.

—*GWV*

To Scott, the heart and soul of my life and work. I love you.
To Ben, Luke, and JP, you're all three my very favorite.
To the HBOS—Hayeses, Olsons, and Singlas—
my best grownup playmates.
To Ayla, for your heart, mind, passion, and gifts
that make the world beautiful.

—*TPB*

Play is often talked about as if
it were a relief from serious learning.
But for children, play is serious learning.
Play is really the work of childhood.

—*Fred Rogers*

CONTENTS

PREFACE

We know what you're thinking: *A book about play? Seriously? Children do that naturally, and I've got bigger fish to fry as a parent—like getting my kids to stop fighting, eat a vegetable every now and then, put down their devices, and give their dolls a bath somewhere other than the toilet.*

We get it.

But many parents—even those of us who are the most intentional and involved with our kids—don't understand the power of play.

Our decades of research and clinical experience with children, along with the burgeoning science of play, has shown us that what adults might view as silly or unimportant is actually the secret language of children. Once we learn that language, we can unlock the best aspects of our children, helping them develop in healthy ways, build skills and confidence, connect better with others, make better choices, and find joy as they become fully themselves.

The good news is, you don't have to be a professional play therapist to understand and help support your kids' play. It doesn't require expensive toys or hours of time. In fact, all it takes is your participation: By spending just a few minutes playing with your child on a regular basis, you can significantly amplify the developmental, relational, and neurological benefits they receive from activities they already find joyful and effortless.

Wait, so you're talking about me actually joining in the play?

Yes. Your participation in your child's play is what makes the difference. You've probably heard experts talk about the importance of play for kids, and you might have even read books about it. But this parent-participatory approach is different, and it has the power to pay huge dividends in your child's growth and development, and in your relationship with them. We call it the PlayStrong approach. And in this book we're going to show you not only *why* it's so effective but also exactly *how* to do it through seven simple strategies.

Let's break it down for you, beginning with three big ideas about play:

Point #1: Play is in children's nature.

Before children can talk, they live their thoughts and emotions through their play, and PlayStrong is about being with our kids in that first language, approaching their trials and accomplishments with creativity, joy, and connection. It's what they do best and want to do most. And typically, their favorite type of play is when their parents join in.

Point #2: Play builds crucial skills and reduces unwanted behaviors.

It's good that kids like to play, because by experimenting and accomplishing tasks through the fun of play, children develop confidence, resilience, self-understanding, and other important life skills. With the help of the adults in kids' lives, these abilities then reduce the behaviors that drive parents crazy—fighting, rudeness, tantrums, and so on—since the new skills lead to better self-control, empathy, and other attributes necessary for successful interactions with their world. Any time you need to gain cooperation or handle discipline moments—whether you're trying to get shoes on, or devices off—play can make all the difference.

Point #3: Play gives kids appropriate ways to express and process their emotions.

It's not only through building life skills that play helps children behave better. When kids have the attention of their caregivers and feel seen and understood, their emotions can be released in ways other than exploding into tantrums. Rather than erupting, in other words, the emotions get processed and released in the play. For decades, play therapists have learned to watch for details in children's play that communicate what they're feeling and even when they are struggling in some way. You can learn to do the same, thus helping your kids deal with difficult emotions they may not even be aware of. Even as kids get older, play can act as a crucial second language, allowing parents to break through when other ways of communicating fail. When kids have gone through a difficult experience, play can be a powerful way for them to not just process what has happened but to even *heal* as they play.

Put these three points together, and we end up with some really good news: Consistently playing with our kids—even if for only a few minutes per day—makes them happier; creates an environment for their growth into successful, well-adjusted people; and makes our job easier since it helps kids better control their emotions and bodies.

Let's be honest: Most of us are pretty clueless about *how* to play with our kids and sometimes don't even really enjoy it! We get this. Sure, we may appreciate certain aspects of playing with our kids, but most—virtually all—of us often have moments of dread at the thought of getting on all fours to make toy car sounds or sit in a tiny chair for a tea party. We don't know whether to make the crashing noise or to say "vroom vroom," and we don't know whether to raise our pinky as we take a sip. (We promise: You're not the only one!) Or we're not good at kicking a ball or playing veterinarian. What our kids are doing can feel foreign to us. We're not sure when it's going to end or who's going to clean it all up. And while they want us to play, they're often unhappy with *how* we play—"You're doing it wrong!"—so it can be unpleasant for both adult and child.

Furthermore, because the way our kids play can seem so alien, grown-ups often take too much of the lead, trying to guide activities in ways that make sense to *us*. In doing so, we can short-circuit the process that creates the many powerful benefits play offers. Parent-led play can definitely have its place, but when we follow a child's lead, that's when the real magic happens.

PLAY PROVIDES A WORLD OF BENEFITS.

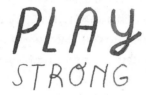

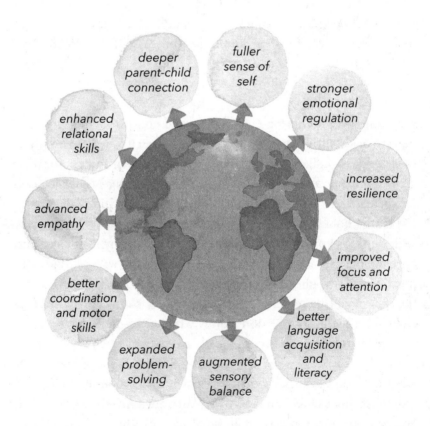

The PlayStrong approach will help you work that magic. We'll show you that it's possible to learn some simple "how to" steps for playing with your kids that will help your whole family reap the benefits and more fully enjoy the times you join your children as they play. We don't think it's a stretch to say that you and your kids will never be the same. Nor will your relationship.

Wondering Whether This Book Is for You?

If you're a perfect parent who never does anything wrong and loves playing constantly with your children, then this book isn't for you. In fact, you don't even exist—because there's no such thing as a perfect parent.

Instead, we're addressing parents and caregivers who are just like us: flawed, busy, well-meaning-but-continuing-to-mess-up humans who often experience a paradoxical set of notions. On one hand we feel that we never have time away from our kids, while on the other we worry that we don't give them *enough* of our time and attention.

This book is for you if you worry about whether your child is developing on a healthy trajectory—or if you feel OK about your kid's development and you just want to optimize it. It's for you if you're worried about some behaviors and emotional dysregulation you see creeping in—or if you just want to give your kids better social emotional intelligence and decision-making skills. It's definitely for you if you want a better relationship with your child—if you want things to be more relaxed and fun, rather than stressful and strained.

Whoever you are as a caregiver right now, the seven PlayStrong strategies we'll offer in the coming pages are designed to meet you *wherever you are.* They'll help you strengthen and deepen your relationship with your child, while enhancing their emotional and behavioral life and expression.

In other words, our starting point is that parents are imperfect and parenting is hard, and that one of the best ways you can make things easier on yourself and your kids is to spend a few minutes each day playing together.

Does that mean that you'll never again lose your temper or say something you regret? Not at all. But the PlayStrong approach does offer us strategies for connecting with our kids even as we remain less-than-perfect caregivers.

And by the way, even though we often use the word "parent" throughout the book, we want you to know that these ideas are intended for any adult who cares for or works with developing children, including teachers, therapists, grandparents, relatives, healthcare workers, coaches, camp counselors, or anyone else doing the important work of supporting kids. Primarily geared toward the years from birth to ten, this approach is especially for grown-ups— *any grown-ups*—who play a nurturing role in the lives of toddlers, school-age children, and preteens.

What's more, the PlayStrong approach is just as powerful with kids who are neurodivergent as it is with those who are neurotypical. It helps parents understand who their child is—their temperament, how their brain is wired, and where their unique child's interests and talents lie. What we'll be teaching in the coming pages is especially transformative for kids who are neurodivergent—who may experience anxiety or overwhelm, including children with sensory processing or attentional challenges, kids on the spectrum, or the highly sensitive, gifted, and 2E (twice-exceptional) kids, and the like.

The same goes for the age of your children. In this book we'll be focusing, for the most part, on parents of babies, toddlers, preschoolers, and school-age children (birth to ten), but really, every kid (teens and even young adults included) can benefit from having parents who give them attention, clue in to their inner world, delight in them, and consistently join with them in playful ways.

Here's What's Coming

In the next chapter we'll introduce you to the principles that guide the PlayStrong approach. Then, each of the book's ensuing chapters will focus on one particular PlayStrong strategy, with each strategy building on the ones that precede it. Our goal is to present the information as simply as possible. We'll briefly explain some theory and research behind the strategy, then quickly move to the practical stuff, breaking it down in simple steps and providing you with lots of examples and illustrations that will help make it all clear. And for each strategy, we'll highlight one main message your child will be able to take away from that approach, along with one primary skill (or set of skills) that the strategy will build in your child.

For example, soon we'll introduce the *Think Out Loud* strategy, where we'll focus on the concept that play allows parents to teach kids about their inner worlds of thoughts, intentions, and emotions. Kids whose parents practice this strategy as they play together will receive the message "Someone understands me, and I can understand myself." And those children will begin taking immediate steps toward developing the skill of understanding and expressing their inner world. (We'll explain this much more fully in the chapter itself.)

The second strategy, *Make Yourself a Mirror,* expands the concept from the previous chapter and focuses on emotional awareness and empathy. We'll show you how to use play to help your child begin to build a deeper understanding of their emotional life, and what that means in their empathetic interactions with others. That self-awareness, and that empathy, are the outcomes this strategy produces. The message they'll receive is "Someone tunes in to me. I can tune in to others."

The third strategy, *Bring Emotions to Life,* takes the first two chapters and expands them in very practical ways, emphasizing steps to help children move from simply becoming aware of their inner worlds to actually understanding, managing, and expressing their emotions. These are the desired outcomes from this strategy, and the message kids will receive is "Someone will help me recognize and make sense of my big feelings."

The fourth strategy, *Dial Intensity Up or Down,* focuses on understanding kids' sensory preferences and responding to our children's struggles based on what they most need in that moment. The highlighted skill in this case is the ability to dial things down when kids become too intense or dial the energy up when they're wanting to withdraw or shut down in some way that's not helpful to them. The message they receive here is "Someone is going to be here for me when I'm out of control and can't handle things very well by myself."

Next comes the fifth strategy, *Scaffold and Stretch,* where we teach you how to inject safe and fun challenges into your play with your child. In doing so, you can help develop focus and resilience, stretching inner and outer skills that will produce mental strength that can be a resource for a lifetime. The message here is "Someone is going to show up for me when things get hard, and I can handle more than I think I can."

The sixth strategy, *Narrate to Integrate,* focuses on an activity— storytelling—with the power to change a mood, an interaction, an expectation, or a seemingly unsolvable situation. We'll look at how narrative in play can help kids learn to resolve problems, handle conflict, and deal with difficult emotions. They'll receive the message "I can use stories to better understand what's going on around me, then make choices that are good for me and that help me take charge of a situation."

The seventh strategy, *Set Playtime Parameters,* addresses a question we get all the time when we teach this material to parents: *What do I do when play gets out of hand?* We'll discuss how best to lovingly and respectfully set appropriate and well-defined boundaries that clearly communicate our expectations, thus giving our kids opportunities to discover new flexibility and adaptable skills they can use to respect the rules of a situation and make positive decisions. The message they'll receive here is "Someone is going to keep me safe and help me learn to do that for myself."

The final PlayStrong strategy involves being playful *Beyond the Playroom.* It makes the argument that you take the concepts and ideas from all the earlier strategies and employ them in ways that don't relate specifically to playtime. We'll talk about the many ways you can use playfulness even when you're not actually playing: to change a mood, to gain compliance, to inject fun into a boring moment, and on and on. When you introduce playfulness and fun into a difficult situation with your child—getting them out of the bathtub, convincing them to go to soccer practice, persuading them to finish their reading, and so on—you not only strengthen your relationship; you also model the idea that conflict is a natural part of relationships and that we can move on from it afterward. And they'll be getting the message that life is fun and joy is a good thing. They will, of course, also learn that life's not always fun and that we all have to do many things we don't actually want to do. But along the way, they'll have the experience that life is to be enjoyed and that, even when we're not getting to do exactly what we want to do, we can still find a way to be happy.

Each strategy offers significant benefits by itself, but the power of the PlayStrong approach is the way the various components build on one another. After reading the short chapter about the first strategy, you'll be ready to begin putting it to use right away. But keep in mind that it's only the first step. So jump in and use it—we'll be specific in showing you how—then as soon as you can, begin adding the other strategies. The more various techniques and strategies you include in your playtime with your kids, the more you'll see huge strides in the approach's overall effectiveness.

One other thing: This isn't an easy "read this book and all your parenting problems will be solved" kind of program. Yes, the strategies are simple to understand. But it's the repeated experiences with your kid that will pay off most significantly. The one idea we most want you to walk away with is this:

Play.

Make a little time for play every day if you can. More important than the amount of time you spend is the *consistency.* Just a few minutes each day will not only help your child develop the skills they need to thrive in this world but also add up to a lifetime of joyful memories about the time you spent together.

The
Way *of* Play

PlayStrong Parenting

At its core, the PlayStrong approach is about just what it sounds like: It uses play to make kids stronger. Stronger in their emotional intelligence. Stronger mentally and cognitively. Stronger in their empathy. Stronger relationally. Even stronger academically. PlayStrong supports positive family connections by enabling shifts toward mindful discipline when kids are showing challenging behavior.

By adopting the techniques and perspectives of PlayStrong, you can radically change your relationship with your children. Through the years working at our institute—the Play Strong Institute in Pasadena, California—we've empowered thousands of caregivers to engage with children in a unique way that truly makes a difference. Parents have learned to use play to help a child move out of a meltdown. Teachers have transformed their lesson plans to become more alive and engaging. Therapists have discovered whole new ways to reach young clients who are resistant to traditional clinical methods. Coaches have discovered new approaches to instill confidence in kids who'd previously hung back on the sidelines. We've seen the PlayStrong techniques work, again and again.

Before we get started with the practical strategies, let's take a few minutes to define some of the key terms and concepts in the PlayStrong approach.

What We Mean When We Talk About "Play"

We're big fans of Little League and dance classes and lots of other types of structured enrichment activities, but that's not what we're talking about here. Instead, we have in mind unstructured, child-led play. We'll explain much more fully in the coming chapters, but the basic idea is that when you spend just a few minutes a day playing with your kids—focusing on them, giving them undivided attention, enjoying being together—something pretty special occurs, for your child, for you, and for your relationship.

The PlayStrong approach is about creating a mindset that focuses on who the child is and what they need. When we play with them, we're not only giving them our attention, we're also getting to know them at a deep level, so we can better understand who they are and how we can bring out the best in them. Play, in other words, is a way of being in relationship. It's a mindset that prioritizes understanding our child and embracing all of their individuality and uniqueness.

> Play is a way of being in relationship. It's a mindset that prioritizes understanding our child and embracing all of their individuality and uniqueness.

Playing with our kids and really getting to know them is a little like scuba diving. From above the surface of the water, it's hard to know what's really happening down there under the waves. But when you take the plunge, you discover this whole other world: dynamic, real, fascinating, beautiful, and full of life.

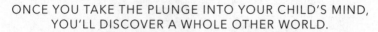

ONCE YOU TAKE THE PLUNGE INTO YOUR CHILD'S MIND, YOU'LL DISCOVER A WHOLE OTHER WORLD.

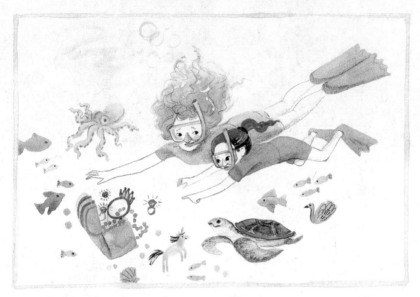

Play lets you take that dive. It offers you the privilege of entering your child's inner life, where you can discover what lights them up, what they feel most deeply about, what upsets them, what they really need, why they do what they do, who they are when they're being totally authentic, and where they can be in perfect harmony with you and everyone around them.

Really, then, *play is a state of mind* where your interactions with your child are full of potential, wisdom, and opportunity. It creates stronger relational connections that allow you to view who they really are, at their essence, and to help them realize so much of the possibility lying within them. Whether you simply join their play for a few minutes, or you use your playful presence to help them deal with a challenging moment they're facing, you're actually playing their phenomenal future self into existence.

YOU'RE NOT JUST PLAYING CARDS. YOU'RE ACTUALLY PLAYING YOUR CHILD'S PHENOMENAL FUTURE SELF INTO EXISTENCE.

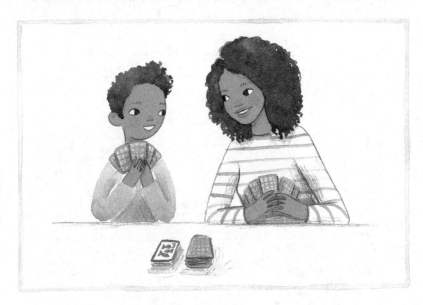

Why Play Is Important
(or, What We Lose When Kids Don't Play)

Play can be integral to a child's relationship with the adults in their life. Likewise, play in general—with parents, with friends, and even alone—is crucial for the development of a child's brain: their curiosity, their language development, their relational skills, their self-image, and on and on. When we don't offer children the opportunity to play on their own terms, we're doing them (and the world) an enormous disservice.

To be blunt, a lack of play stunts their growth.

As only one example, consider education and cognitive development. Play primes a child's brain to become a better learner. In contrast, making kids sit for long stretches at desks and do more table-learning in a typical school day is counterproductive even to the goal of raising test scores or producing more high school graduates.

Play literally makes kids smarter. Studies show better learning outcomes when children are encouraged to take "brain breaks" at school and get more physical outdoor activity. Put differently, we are actually *preventing* kids' academic and cognitive development when we overemphasize screens and technology, and when we replace recess with increased schoolwork and schedule too many after-school hours with activities.

And that's just the cognitive development. We see the same pattern in other domains of a child's maturation. If they're not given the chance to negotiate conflicts with siblings because they're too busy hurrying from one dance lesson to another, they're missing out on important opportunities to learn how to manage their emotions when they're upset. And if they don't have recess or get to play with friends and navigate the complicated playground politics that crop up when adults aren't around, they'll lose those chances to develop the social skills they'll need as they approach and enter adulthood. If they don't have time for free, open play on their own, they miss out on discovering the world, testing and problem-solving, having inner dialogues, and learning about who they are and the incredible power of their own ideas and minds.

So yes, play really is that important—and not only now, but far into the future.

Play's Role as Your Child Grows Up

Speaking of far into the future: If you think about the kind of relationship you want to have when your child is a teenager, then a young adult, what comes to mind? We're guessing you'd say that you want them to feel connected to you. That they're willing to come to you in significant moments in their lives—whether they're hurting or celebrating.

And guess what patterns are set up when you play with your child, even when they're very young? Yup—the very dynamics you hope will be there when your child grows into adulthood. By connecting with your child now, you establish the pattern, and the expectation, that a parent-child relationship is one where the two parties know and can count on each other.

When they're a teenager and young adult, our kid obviously won't play the same way they do now. But if they've spent their whole life knowing that we're there for them, that we *get* them in a deep way, that we join with them and pay attention when they tell us something that's important to them—if this is the relational pattern that's been set up all along the way—then that will be the expectation when they're older as well.

When they experience their first breakup or don't get the job they interviewed for and believe they deserve, or when they make the varsity team or get that job, if they've grown up knowing that you're a constant, intentional, clued-in part of their life, then it's much more likely that that expectation will remain as the years roll by. And one of the most powerful ways you can set that expectation is by learning to play again.

> If our kid has spent their whole life knowing that we're there for them, that we *get* them in a deep way, that we join with them and pay attention when they tell us something that's important to them—if this is the relational pattern that's been set up all along the way—then that will be the expectation when they're older as well.

But Don't We All Know How to Play?

To a surprising extent, no, we really don't. The fact is that many parents have no actual idea how to enter the powerful, beautiful, and often foreign world of children's play. It's analogous to breastfeeding. Some new moms think it'll be easy and just "happen" because "it's natural," but many first-time mothers need help and practice to figure out that process, and for many, it's not intuitive at all.

Play is like that. We can try to make it work for a while in certain situations, but many of us simply don't know how to play like children do.

It's not our fault. Our brains have grown and changed since we were children, to the extent that what our kids are doing as they "make a magic potion" or "play bad guys" no longer really makes sense to us. The most natural and fun activities in the world for our child can seem really boring to us.

At least at first.

SOMETIMES WE JUST DON'T KNOW HOW TO PLAY.

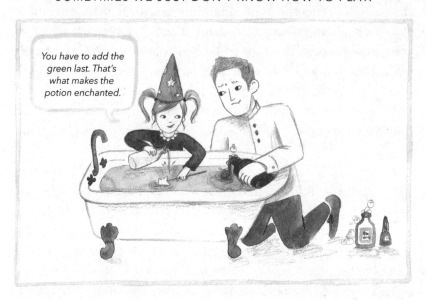

We might assume we know how to play simply because we used to do it so naturally. But actually, our brains don't work that way anymore. We have to relearn what it means to think and play like a child so we can join our kids in the mysterious magic taking place within their powerful but still-developing brain.

So to answer the question, we really can be clueless about how to play—your authors included.

We might assume we know how to play simply because we used to do it so naturally. But actually, our brains don't work that way anymore. We have to relearn what it means to think and play like a child.

Play Improves Kids' Behavior

As we said in the preface, one of the best reasons to play with your kids is that it cuts down on discipline problems. And remember, we're not talking about playing for hours. We mean it when we say that if you can do it for just a few minutes each day, or even most days, you and your child will both reap huge rewards. You'll likely both be happier, and you can rest assured that not only will you be advancing your child's cognitive, emotional, and relational development, but yes, you'll see fewer unwanted behaviors as well.

To say that differently: One huge advantage of the PlayStrong approach is that it makes parenting so much easier. When kids have the attention of their caregivers and feel seen and understood, their emotions can be released in ways other than exploding into tantrums. Rather than erupting, in other words, the emotions get taken care of in the play.

This is called "responsive play," since it involves kids *responding* to stimuli and their environment. Responsive play allows them to largely bypass much of the misbehavior that might otherwise result from pent-up emotions, because those emotions are being channeled and expressed through the activity of play. Especially as kids get older, play can become a second language through which parents can relate to them, reading their emotions and learning how best to elicit appropriate responses to situations.

One huge advantage of the PlayStrong approach is that it makes parenting so much easier. When kids have the attention of their caregivers and feel seen and understood, their emotions can be released in ways other than exploding into tantrums. Rather than erupting, in other words, the emotions get taken care of in the play.

Another type of play, "preventative play," is a more proactive (rather than responsive) activity. It focuses on building skills and developing abilities *beforehand* so that kids can better manage their body and emotions in a heated moment. We'll discuss lots of examples of preventative play in the coming chapters, showing how you can, for example, create dramatic or challenging situations to help build strength and resilience. The characteristics that result from preventative play—flexibility, grit, confidence, empathy, self-understanding, and other important life skills—can lower a child's overall stress and anxiety, meaning that certain problematic behaviors never crop up in the first place. Instead, the child can exercise better self-control and deepen their understanding of others, leading to more successful interactions with their world.

None of this means, by the way, that you should be permissive when it comes to your kids' behavior. The science is clear that children experience the best outcomes when parents set boundaries and limits *while also* offering relational connection. We're big on the importance of parents communicating clear expectations and setting well-defined boundaries; that's how kids know what the rules are, and that helps them feel safe. *And* it's possible, and even important, that parents communicate love and support alongside that limit setting.

Notice, too, that when we join our kids in play, we're actually doing so much more than killing time. We are creating the opportunity for our children to grow into competent, self-aware, inner-directed, secure, peaceful, loving individuals. This makes parenting easier, in both the short and long term.

There is no particular "right time" to play: It's up to you. Head to the park after school and see what happens there. Set a timer and see how fast everyone can get dressed if it helps make the morning routine go more smoothly. Wrestle and roughhouse together after dinner if it changes a mood and reduces bedtime conflict—or even just for fun. If you'd like, plan out specific moments to be exclusively present and focused on your child. Or, just as good, use any of the many interactions you share over the course of a day—in the car or standing in line at a store—as opportunities to play and help them become the calm listener, cooperative problem solver, and respectful communicator you've always wanted them to be.

Can you communicate your love and all the lessons you want to teach without ever getting on the floor with your child and playing with them? Yes, of course. There are a multitude of ways parents can show up for their kids and give them what they need, and we encourage you to use everything at your disposal. But why would you neglect using kids' first language, play, as one of your primary tools?

Our brains are different from our kids' brains, and what we're doing when we play with them is entering their worlds using their language to interact with them in a deeper and more significant way, one that comes absolutely naturally to them. The key idea of the PlayStrong approach is that by spending time with your child and really giving them your attention, you'll become clearer than ever before, in any given situation, about what's going on in the mind of your child and what they need from you to be more thoughtfully engaged in daily routines, family activities, and important tasks. Simply by taking a few minutes here and there throughout the day!

By spending time with your child and really giving them your attention, you'll become clearer than ever before, in any given situation, about what's going on in the mind of your child and what they need from you to be more thoughtfully engaged in daily routines, family activities, and important tasks. Simply by taking a few minutes here and there throughout the day!

Think Out Loud

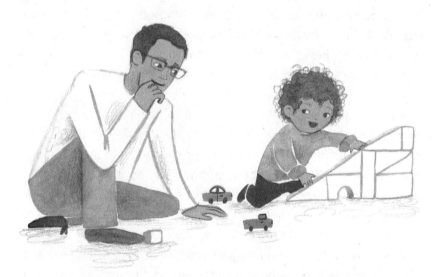

Primary skill being developed in the child:
Awareness of their inner world: thoughts, feelings, wishes, intentions, and more.

Primary message received by the child:
Someone understands me, and I can understand myself.

At times it seemed that Theo hated his baby sister. From the first moment he laid eyes on little Emma, so many of his actions screamed, "You're the enemy!"

When he hid her favorite hippo, she cried. When he pinched her legs at the park, she screamed. And when he swiped her smoothie, pouring it all over the kitchen floor, he laughed while the family dog lapped it up. As he grew older, the conflict only intensified.

Playtime for five-year-old Theo and two-year-old Emma was often a complete disaster. Theo would want to build with his blocks, and Emma would try to join in. But as soon as she got close, Theo would scream in her face or push her over. Once he ran across the room to tackle her, like a linebacker plowing into a quarterback. He was so fast that Kevin, his father, couldn't get there in time to block him.

Kevin was a single dad, and he tried everything he could think of: bribes, threats, punishments, timeouts. But nothing worked. He felt exasperated because he couldn't figure out how to help his young son handle himself better and be kinder to his sister. He didn't want to spend these precious early years breaking up fights and repeatedly sending his children to their separate corners.

Nagging questions and doubts began to materialize in his mind: *Should it be this hard for my children to play together? Is this typical, or is there something wrong with my son?* He wanted to teach his children important life skills about communication and compromise, relationships and resilience, but he worried that all he was doing was constantly refereeing their fights so they could all simply survive until bedtime. And even that wasn't going so well.

Does any of this sound familiar? Are there times when your kids get stuck in a behavior and you can't figure out how to get them out of it? Maybe it's sibling conflict like Kevin was facing with his kids, or maybe it's about screen time, emotional issues, school difficulties, or something else. Unless your family is very, very unusual, you and your kids are facing an issue or two (or nine!) that you feel like you just can't get on top of. This is where the first PlayStrong strategy, Think Out Loud, comes in. It'll take time and consistency, but it can be the key to resolving many of the difficult issues you and your family regularly face.

What we're offering here is a different perspective on handling conflict, one that lays the groundwork *ahead of time* and that's also responsive to children's overwhelming needs *in the moment*. It's a way to make your child more aware of the source of their frustration and more willing to observe their own powerful needs and drives. Over time they'll be better—not perfect, but better—at expressing their thoughts and feelings to others in a balanced and productive manner. Let's talk about how to do that.

What we're offering here is a different perspective on handling conflict, one that lays the groundwork *ahead of time* and that's also responsive to children's overwhelming needs *in the moment*. It's a way to make your child more aware of the source of their frustration and more willing to observe their own powerful needs and drives. Then, they'll be better—not perfect, but better—at expressing their thoughts and feelings to others in a balanced and productive manner.

Think Out Loud: The Strategy

When children automatically react to a negative situation, they're largely acting without thinking, driven by overwhelming impulses bubbling up from the more primitive parts of their brain. Unless they have trustworthy, reliable adults who can step in and help regulate emotions and behaviors without getting too overwhelmed themselves, kids will repeat their angry reactions so often that those behaviors, or temporary *states,* begin to look more like long-lasting negative habits and even become *traits.*

The good news is that there's a way we can help develop our children's ability to regulate themselves through the power of self-awareness. The more you can cultivate this skill in your kids, the more they can avoid losing control of their emotions (and bodies and minds) when things don't go their way. That's what we'll be aiming for in the first few chapters of this book.

Thinking out loud is the first step to teaching kids to pay attention to what's happening inside themselves so they can develop positive, conscious, intentional *responses,* instead of intense and off-the-cuff *reactions.* With practice and our help, kids really can develop a fuller awareness of what's going on inside their minds. And that awareness can grow stronger and stronger over the years as your child moves through adolescence and eventually becomes an adult.

Think about what a difference it would've made for Theo if he'd had this skill at the ready whenever he became upset with Emma. If only he could *observe* what was going on inside his own mind *before* he lashed out at his sister, he could make a different choice. If only he could develop this one powerful observational skill, then his father could work with him on applying it in his interactions with his sister as he matured until eventually he could regulate his behaviors on his own.

This is where thinking out loud comes in. What we're doing, essentially, is introducing our kids to their inner world. We play with them, and while doing so, we help them become more conscious of their own thoughts, feelings, plans, ideas, wishes, and intentions.

> What we're doing, essentially, is introducing our kids to their inner world. We play with them, and while doing so, we help them become more conscious of their own thoughts, feelings, plans, ideas, wishes, and intentions.

Sounds logical enough, but here's the challenge: Kids aren't born knowing what they think and feel. In fact, young children especially don't even know what a "thought" or "feeling" (or "sensation," "intention," or "motivation") is until they learn it, when development unfolds to allow that sophisticated process to happen. As spoken language develops, typically somewhere between a child's first and second birthday, they begin to express their thoughts and feelings in words because they've spent a lot of time watching us do it.

But they can still struggle.

As kids get older, as often as we ask them to "use your words" and express themselves, they often haven't developed the neural connectivity or the necessary skills yet, or they're too dysregulated to access them. If they could find the right words in the moment, they would use them—but so often they can't.

Instead, while we work with them on developing the ability to express themselves in words, we have to tune in and interpret their actions. There's a phrase we like that you'll already know if you read Tina's book with Dan Siegel, *No-Drama Discipline:* "Behavior is communication." Kids' actions tell a story. With their behavior, they show us the very lessons they need to be taught and the skills they need to learn. So we want to view all behavior as communication, then get curious about what it is that's causing that behavior.

Sure, Kevin would have loved for Theo's response, when his sister encroached on his block stacking, to be, "I'm feeling very angry, so I'd better watch myself and make good decisions." But at Theo's level of development, that kind of emotional-linguistic response was far beyond his reach, especially in the heat of the moment. This kind of emotionally aware language is hard even for mature adults!

So what *was* Theo communicating?

That he lacked the skill of self-awareness—the first step toward controlling his own actions. That's what his behavior was telling his father.

All kids, in fact, need to build the same skills. That's why the focus of the first PlayStrong strategy is to cultivate a level of self-awareness in children. We want to introduce them to their inner world so

BEHAVIOR IS COMMUNICATION.

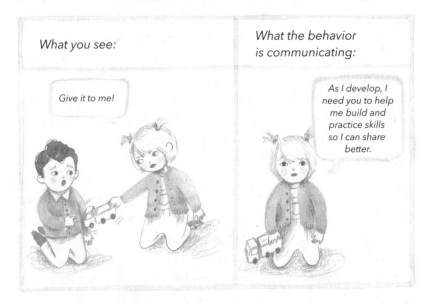

they can pay attention to what's going on with their thoughts and emotions, then make better choices as they mature and grow up. They won't get it right away, of course, but you know that old proverb about the journey of a thousand miles beginning with the first step? Introducing self-awareness, even at a rudimentary level, is the first step in the thousand-mile journey toward self-regulation and healthy development.

Think Out Loud: Step by Step

You've seen what happens when you've watched your kids play. Right now, imagine your child's face when they're about to begin drawing, or creating something out of assorted Legos, or building a world full of action figures or dolls. Can you picture that distinct facial expression? The classic "I'm thinking" look, as if their eyes are scanning the air about a foot away, searching for a great idea? Then, within a few seconds, their facial expression brightens. They might even give out a little gasp of excitement, then pick up the first objects they'll use. Then their face takes on an entirely different look. Maybe their tongue appears at the corner of their mouth and their eyes squint a little.

What you're seeing is a look of intense concentration as they begin to take the idea from the thinking stage into direct action. You're witnessing the birth of an idea from what we might call "the brain lab." Imagine the laboratory of a brilliant scientist, with a whole team of minions scuttling around performing wild experiments—beakers bubbling, sparks flying, music blaring—and nobody cares when something spills or breaks or blows up, because glorious discoveries are being churned out faster than you can say "Neil deGrasse Tyson." Welcome to your child's brain lab! Think of it like the research and development department of a multilevel high-tech start-up company. It's all about ideas and testing new possibilities.

Something magical is occurring, and this is the time that we want to engage with our kids, helping them notice what's going on within themselves. The overall idea is that we can play with our kids in ways that help them think more fully about what their minds are doing. As we play with them, we observe and then narrate what we see. In doing so, we model for them what it looks like to notice mental and emotional states so that they can perform that type of observation for themselves. Here's how it works, step by step.

> As we play with our kids, we observe and then narrate what we see. In doing so, we model for them what it looks like to observe mental and emotional states so that they can perform that type of observation for themselves.

Step 1: Observe and attune

That brain-lab energy is what you want to tap into. As your child sets up the play scene, you begin by just watching what's going on, listening for clues that allow you to tune in to your child's world. That's all you have to do at the beginning: just observe and listen. This is called attunement, and as you'll soon see, each of the PlayStrong strategies begins with this crucial first step.

There's nothing specific or precise you need to do or think about. Your job is simply to really clue in to what's going on in your child's mind in that moment. Then, once you do that, you're going to be ready to move to the more practical steps.

Step 2: Come up with a hypothesis

In the case of Kevin and Theo, those practical steps might begin with Kevin finding an activity that Emma can busy herself with, then looking for how best to join in as Theo plays with his beloved blocks. At that point Theo's brain lab would likely be clicking into high gear, and soon he'd be creating.

As he did, Kevin would simply watch, noticing what Theo's actions might communicate. As Theo builds his tower, with a ramp leading to it, Kevin would explore interpretations of where things were headed, soon coming up with a hypothesis.

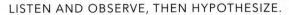

LISTEN AND OBSERVE, THEN HYPOTHESIZE.

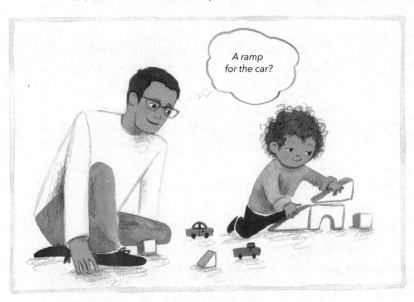

Step 3: Say it out loud

Once you have a hypothesis, try it out. Show your child what it looks like when you tune in to their mind. And don't worry: The simpler the better at this point. You're not getting into any deep thoughts or making any grand pronouncements. Just narrate what you see happening, especially with an eye toward describing your child's mind and intentions.

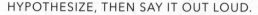

HYPOTHESIZE, THEN SAY IT OUT LOUD.

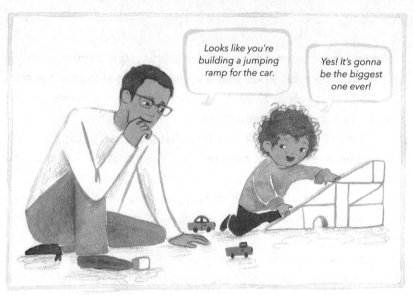

In this interaction, something subtle but significant is taking place. When Kevin correctly guesses Theo's architectural intent, he does much more than just get the right answer. In effect, he connects with his young son about this one fact, which, in this particular moment, is one of the most important elements in Theo's whole world. His dad has understood him. He *gets* him. He sees his mind. Theo, of course, wouldn't put it this way and in all likelihood wouldn't see this moment as even noteworthy. Still, when this type of connection is consistently repeated in playtime interactions day after day, Theo will slowly and increasingly accept—deep down in the core of his being—that his father truly understands who his son is and what matters to him.

> When this type of connection is consistently repeated in playtime interactions day after day, Theo will slowly and increasingly accept—deep down in the core of his being—that his father truly understands who his son is and what matters to him.

Beyond the relational connection, the other significant occurrence here is that Theo gets to see that it's possible for one person to ascertain what's going on in another's mind. Again, he won't consider this fact on a conscious level, and it won't make a huge change right away. But when his dad accurately names that Theo is building a ramp, Theo receives the subtle message that it's possible to understand another person's intentions just by paying attention to what the person is doing. For a child, it's an immense gift when a parent helps them connect language with an awareness of their thoughts, feelings, and actions.

Right now you might be thinking that we're making too big a deal of this one comment—*Looks like you're building a jumping ramp for the car*—but again, when combined with numerous other similar interactions, Theo will grow up knowing that he and his father are closely connected and that his dad pays attention to, and yes, understands, what's going on in his mind.

These messages are reinforced during each interaction when Kevin and his son spend a few more minutes together with the blocks. (Remember—only a few minutes a day can have a *huge* impact!) Kevin simply works through the three steps, again and again. He continues to observe and listen. He forms a hypothesis. Then he says it out loud. Rinse and repeat.

Again, this isn't rocket science (even though the car *is* flying), and there's no mysterious phraseology you have to learn if you want to interact with your kids in this way. Notice what Kevin's doing here.

LISTEN AND OBSERVE, HYPOTHESIZE, THEN SAY IT OUT LOUD.

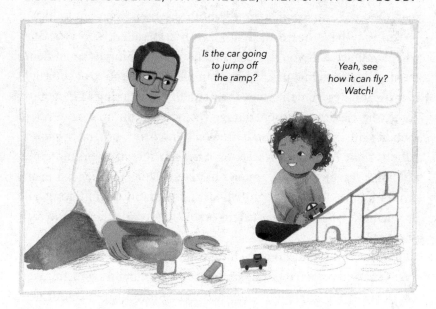

LISTEN AND OBSERVE, HYPOTHESIZE, THEN SAY IT OUT LOUD.

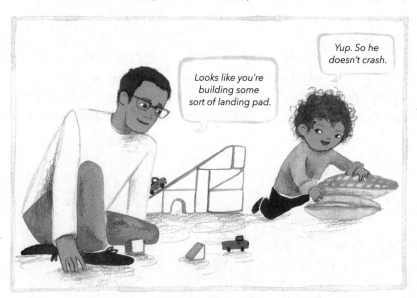

He's simply perceiving what Theo is doing, then narrating what he sees. Observe and listen, form a hypothesis, then say it out loud.

You may have heard of a similar process called "sportscasting," where you act as if you're a commentator describing to an audience the details of a game on TV. For example, a preschool teacher might narrate and describe the steps their students are taking as they move about the classroom to encourage the acquisition of new developmental skills: *Oh, you found a little pair of scissors,* or, *You're going to cut out some circles.* Sportscasting has been shown to promote pre-academic learning in the context of play, such as language, fine and gross motor skills, and cognitive tasks like planning, initiating, and problem-solving. Sportscasting is fantastic for kids during the early years.

But the Think Out Loud technique goes further. Your goal here is to do more than narrate the simple actions of babies and toddlers. This PlayStrong strategy is intended to begin to introduce our children to their inner world, so we need to look more closely and go beyond basic descriptions, showing that we can connect with our kids' *intentions, wishes, and motivations,* not just what we can see on the surface of things.

That's why actually speaking aloud your hypothesis is so key—you're paying attention to not just your child's behavior but also their feelings, desires, impulses, plans, thoughts, and on and on—all of the various activities of their *mind.* You're noticing all of these facets of their being, and you're "thinking them out loud."

> You're paying attention to not just your child's behavior but also their feelings, desires, impulses, plans, thoughts, and on and on—all of the various activities of their *mind.* You're noticing all of these facets of their being, and you're "thinking them out loud."

Before the age of three, small children really enjoy sportscasting, because they love our attention and want to soak up anything positive we have to say about their activities. But as kids get older, they want to interact with others using more abstract thinking and complexity, and they start to get wise to adults who carry on with basic sportscasting. *Yes, I already told you I wanted to use the scissors. Why do you keep repeating whatever I say?* Thinking out loud is therefore a step up in sophistication, the next level of sportscasting for children as they mature.

By the way, as you practice this strategy, you won't hit on a correct hypothesis every time. And that's not a problem for most kids. In fact, it can be beneficial to the whole process, since even when you guess wrong once in a while, it gives you and your child one more way to interact, and they're happy to correct you!

Really, as long as you just continue narrating what you notice, following your child's cues, there's not much you can do wrong. The only real mistake you can make is to take charge, for instance, by giving commands, correcting your child, or questioning their decisions.

DON'T WORRY WHEN YOU GUESS WRONG.

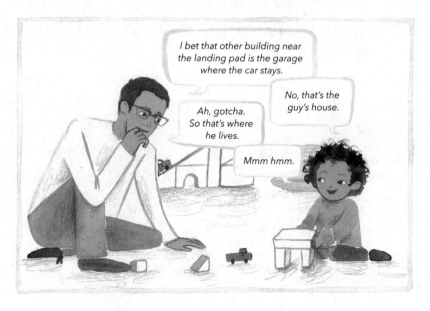

WHAT NOT TO DO: COMMAND.

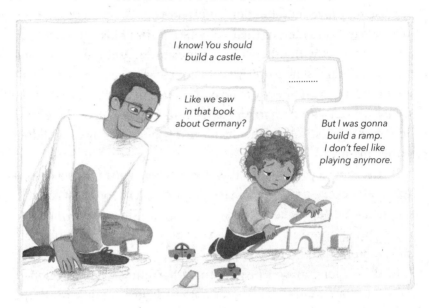

WHAT NOT TO DO: CORRECT.

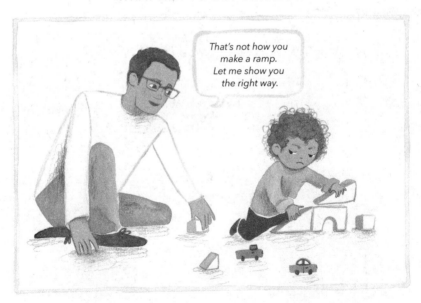

WHAT NOT TO DO: QUESTION.

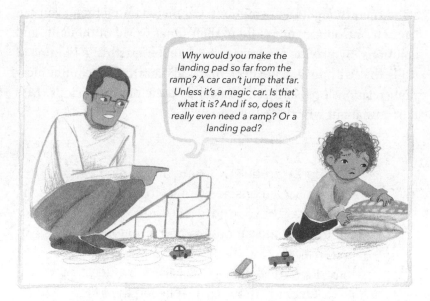

Aside from taking over, you almost can't mess this up. Just notice what's happening and follow along, describing what you see going on in your child's mind and in their intentions. When Theo repeatedly experiences his father joining with him in this way, accurately anticipating and recognizing the contents of his mind, he'll gradually begin to understand that it's possible for one person to look into another person's mind and at least guess what might be going on in there. He'll also be more engaged with his dad and more eager to share his thoughts and feelings as well.

Now you might have another objection: *That's all well and good, that Theo is gaining self-awareness and getting to connect with his father and all. But that's not going to keep him from going ballistic the next time his sister shows up and destroys his carefully constructed ramp-and-landing-pad mechanism.*

No, it's not. At least, not right away. Again, we're talking about a process over time, one that requires many reps before it bears fruit. But an important foundation is being laid when that ramp is built, and when the next day a train station is created, and the next day a soccer ball is passed right where the other player is going. Simply by regularly taking a few minutes to make a conscious effort to see into the motives and intentions of your child, showing you understand their thoughts and emotions and then naming them, you can begin to introduce your child to their inner world of thoughts and emotions. By playing the long game, you'll unearth a gold mine of skills that will positively affect your kid's awareness, communication, relationships, and self-control as their brain develops. Let's talk now about why that's the case.

> Simply by regularly taking a few minutes to make a conscious effort to see into the motives of your child, showing you understand their thoughts and emotions and then naming them, you can begin to introduce your child to their inner world of thoughts and emotions. By playing the long game, you'll unearth a gold mine of skills that will positively affect your kid's awareness, communication, relationships, and self-control as their brain develops.

The Reflective Pause

During this time you spend playing with your child, you two are both improving your skills in one key area: reflection. Pausing to reflect is one of the most important parenting abilities to cultivate, because it invites us to slow down and catch our breath so we, ourselves, can think before reacting—just as we want our children to do. A big reason that a reflective pause is so important, of course, is that we want to be able to stop and think when we're upset, and avoid saying or doing something we wish we hadn't. But more to the point here, reflection has a lot to do with how we look at and feel about our kids, as well as our ability to guide our kids toward meaningful solutions.

For example, if Kevin had looked at Theo's behavior and offered a snap judgment about his son, labeling him as "stubborn" or "reckless," or as someone who simply can't get along with his sister, then Kevin would have had a harder time moving past that mental image so that he could work with Theo to build the relational skills he was lacking. And not surprisingly, Theo's behavioral patterns would likely have become predictable, repetitive, and stuck as he continued repeating those unwanted behaviors.

On the other hand, if Kevin, the most caring adult in Theo's life, the one who knows his son better than anyone, could instead choose to see Theo as having thoughts and emotions full of depth and complexity, then he could move beyond overly simplistic caricatures based on snap judgments. Then, from this fuller and deeper perspective, Kevin could respond to his thoughts and feelings with more intention and purpose.

And what about Theo? How would he be affected by the time he spent playing with his father and hearing Kevin hypothesize and narrate what he was thinking and feeling as he played?

Well, there would be a few results. First, he'd know that his dad is someone who engages with him—who shows interest in what Theo cares about and enjoys spending time with him.

Second, he'd gradually begin to comprehend that it's possible to know someone else's mind to some extent. Through repeated interactions as he grew up, he'd learn implicitly that by spending time with another person and paying attention to their thoughts, feelings, and intentions, you can gain a basic sense of what's going on inside their mind.

Then there's not a huge leap to the third result, the primary skill we're shooting for in this first PlayStrong strategy: that Theo would be introduced to the existence of his own internal world. He'd learn, in other words, that it's possible to pay attention to what's happening not just inside the mind of another but also within *his own* mind. Theo won't be able to fully comprehend the concept of self-reflection for several years, but still, he's getting prepared to understand, at a deep level, that it's possible to observe and respond to what's happening within himself. Kevin can make the process more and more explicit along the way, consistently helping him "think about his thinking" and "pay attention to his feelings" so that Theo learns to watch for what's going on in his mind and make better decisions based on what he discovers.

With this skill as a part of his way of interacting with the world, then, he can much more effectively choose, with intention and purpose, how he responds to various situations he faces. After all, if he's able to pay attention to and even somewhat understand his own thoughts and feelings, intentions and motivations, then it stands to reason that he can allow his observations to guide his actions. And that means that over the months and years, sudden, reactive outbursts will become much less frequent. Those unthinking *reactions,* then, will be replaced, much more frequently, by conscious and intentional *choices* about how he behaves when strong feelings crop up within him.

WHAT THINKING OUT LOUD DOES FOR A KID.

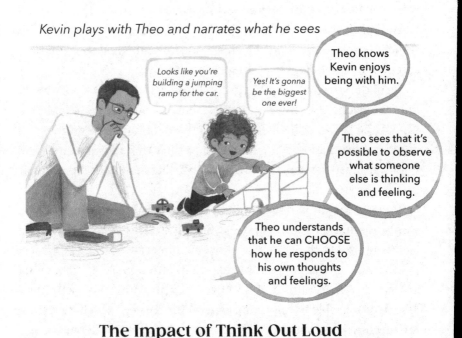

Kevin plays with Theo and narrates what he sees

The Impact of Think Out Loud

What does this mean, practically, the next time Theo sees Emma moving toward his newest creation? Well, it's not going to keep him from feeling annoyed, or even angry. He's still five, after all, and she's still his little sister. She's going to want to involve herself in his activity, and it's going to drive him crazy when she does. And over and over again, he's still going to want to react out of his anger.

But slowly, over time, the entire process can begin to evolve into a completely different interaction. With repetition, and with his father's help, Theo can become more and more proficient at noticing the fury boiling up within him. And that's the crucial step, because once he can notice his emotions, he won't be nearly as much at their mercy. If he can simply *notice* what's happening inside himself, he can at least begin to handle himself with more control. Again, he'll need plenty of practice, and lots of support from his father, who can make the lesson more explicit along the way.

One skill like this can be a real game changer—and not just for Theo and his dad. Think about how different Emma's early years will be if she has a brother with even an ounce of self-reflection. Not only will she get yelled at less often, but just as important, she'll now have a healthy model to look up to. And of course, Kevin will play with his young daughter along the way as well, just as he does with his son, narrating what he sees and helping her learn the art of self-reflection.

Isn't it exciting to think about what this kind of change could mean to a family, both now and into the future? Look at the way the simple act of playing with your kids for only a few minutes a day can set the stage for calmer interactions, more self-control, better sibling interactions, stronger parent-child relationships, and on and on. Then think about how different they'll be in the future, as they develop into tweens and teens who interact with the world from a place of self-awareness and with an ability to pause and *decide* how to respond to a situation, rather than just automatically flying off the handle.

Go one step further: Think about what kind of parents they'll be if by the time they reach adulthood they have a couple of decades of developing these intra- and interpersonal skills. The benefits go on, literally, in an infinite fashion. Now we're *really* talking about playing the long game.

As we close this first chapter, let's be clear: This is just the first strategy. It's pretty powerful on its own, and you can put it into practice right away. But in the next chapter we're going to teach you another, related, strategy, and when you put the two together during your playtime with your kids, you'll begin to see even larger and more significant benefits. Then as you add each subsequent strategy to the mix, you'll be building a whole set of skills and capabilities in your children that will help them become the kind of smart, caring, relational, well-balanced kids you want to raise. That's when you'll have a real sense of what we mean when we talk about the genius of play.

Make Yourself a Mirror

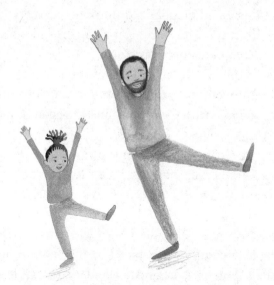

Primary skill being developed in the child:
A deeper understanding of their own emotional life, which can
deepen their connection with and empathy for others.

Primary message received by the child:
Someone tunes in to me. I can tune in to others.

Now that you have one strategy to begin using right away, let's talk about another easy one that will help you keep working toward developing within your kids the self-reflection and relational skills that will benefit them throughout their lives. None of these strategies by themselves will give children all that they need in life, nor will they remove all the hard stuff from parenting. But as you add each new PlayStrong strategy to your overall parenting approach, you'll begin to notice significant growth in your kids and in your relationships with them.

This second PlayStrong strategy emphasizes building some of the same skills and capabilities in your kids that the first one did. But whereas the first strategy focused on using your *words* to move your children toward developing the skills they need, this second one is about how you can use your *physical presence* to do the same. And while Think Out Loud emphasized introducing kids to their inner worlds, this strategy—Make Yourself a Mirror—focuses more specifically on helping kids develop empathy by better understanding their own emotions. The basic idea is that you watch for ways to mirror the actions of your kids, thus communicating how tuned in you are to them. You join with them, relationally—again, simply by playing together.

Not long ago, Georgie met in her office with Annie, a concerned and frustrated mother of a nine-year-old. Georgie could tell from the way Annie was biting her lip that she was afraid to ask what might be going on for her youngest child, Chloe. She explained to Georgie, "I read somewhere that every child is born with empathy. I think most kids are probably naturally capable of caring about others' feelings, but my husband and I are starting to wonder about Chloe." The mom of three could easily think of something sweet her older children had done for someone lately, like make a card for Grandma after a minor medical procedure, but Chloe had to be pushed and prodded. She rarely came up with kind gestures on her own.

Finally, she spoke. "I know Chloe cares about our family," Annie said, "but maybe she doesn't know how to show it when the stakes are high." Annie spoke about her family's Friday-night tradition called "Mac-opoly": First they'd have helpings of Mom's famous mac and cheese, followed by what was supposed to be a fun round of the classic board game Monopoly. But it rarely turned out to be fun at all. Chloe didn't like to lose. She argued, cheated, and stole the pretend money, regardless of how it affected the other players at the table. She gloated when she won and pouted when she lost. And it was the same at school, where she often got in trouble not only for being too competitive but also for taking seemingly no care about how her words might make her classmates feel. Kids were beginning to avoid playing with her.

Annie felt that she must be the only parent in the world to have such concerns about her daughter, but as Georgie explained, *many* caregivers wonder from time to time whether their kids are fully capable of empathy. An eight-month-old keeps reaching out and pulling a stray tendril of his mother's hair, even though she winces in pain. A giggling three-year-old chases the cat around the house, squealing as she almost catches the skittish kitty by the tail. A fifth grader comes home in tears because her group of "besties" chatted about weekend plans that don't include her. How can these kids be so callous? Do some children simply need to work on flexing their empathy muscles, or could they be missing that muscle altogether? That's just what Annie was wondering about Chloe, and she was worried.

> Do some children simply need to work on flexing their empathy muscles, or could they be missing that muscle altogether?

Diving Deeper into Empathy

Remember what we said in the previous chapter: Behavior is communication. When kids are behaving in ways that make life hard for themselves and those around them, they're simply communicating with us. Screaming, crying, protesting, pouting, whining, arguing, shutting down: All of these actions can be indicators that our kids are having a hard time and that they can really benefit from skill building in certain areas as development unfolds. In Chloe's case, she needed help in developing her empathy skills so she could both notice and then gain a fuller perspective on how her words and actions affected the people around her.

If we're interested in showing kids like Chloe how to consider another person's feelings, both within the home and outside of it, we should discuss some basic terminology around the concept of empathy. Emotion researchers generally define empathy as the ability to sense other people's emotions, coupled with the ability to mentalize, or imagine, what someone else might be thinking or feeling. This basically means that a big part of empathy, or what the research calls "cognitive empathy," is being able to consider how someone else thinks and feels, something we collectively refer to as "putting yourself in another person's shoes." We're not sure who came up with that old saying, but it would be more accurate to say that empathy allows us to think about and try to feel what's going on in someone else's *mind*. The first strategy you read about, Think Out Loud, is all about building more cognitive empathy—between you and your child, and between your child and others—because it allows us to extend thoughtful consideration and reflection about what might be going on in the minds of others.

The other important part of empathy, though, something researchers have termed "affective empathy," proceeds from the sensations and feelings we get in our bodies as a response to others' emotions.

It's one thing to be able to say, "That person's facial expression looks sad, so it's obvious they must feel sad," which is a function of our cognitive empathy. This is typically how preschoolers are taught to identify their own feeling states, by looking at and pointing to charts with drawings of "feeling faces." That's cognitive empathy, and it's an important skill for children (and adults!) to have at their disposal.

But affective empathy goes much deeper. It's about seeing another person crying and then not just noticing but actually *feeling* with

TWO TYPES OF EMPATHY.

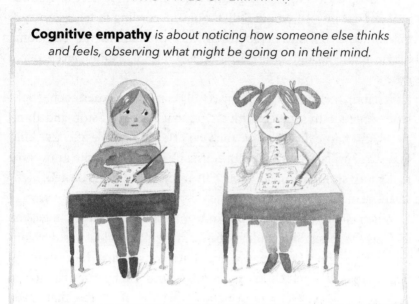

Cognitive empathy *is about noticing how someone else thinks and feels, observing what might be going on in their mind.*

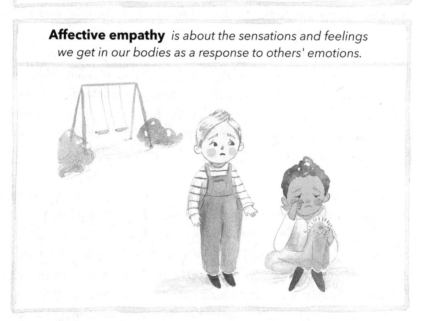

Affective empathy *is about the sensations and feelings we get in our bodies as a response to others' emotions.*

them, sharing in the felt emotion. Chloe could readily say that she loved her family and cared about her friends, but what was most challenging for her was being able to switch on her inner sensors for other people's feelings, particularly when her competitive streak was brought out by a situation. Still, though, according to her mom, seeing someone fall and scrape their knee or watching an emotional movie scene would give Chloe pause, and she might even cry a little.

What that tells us is that she was fully capable of experiencing both types of empathy: the cognitive type that makes us stop and think about and name the other person's experience, and the affective kind that stirs similar emotions within us. She just didn't quite know how to do both simultaneously, especially in the middle of a heated, high-stakes game of Monopoly.

When Georgie explained this information, Annie gave a huge, visible sigh of relief. She could stop worrying that Chloe was developmentally lagging in empathy and start considering more hopeful possibilities for her child's emerging social capabilities. It helped even more when Georgie explained that the attributes that made Chloe good at *competing* were also evidence that she could *cooperate* as well. The two activities might seem like opposites, but they work from many of the same fundamental skills. Both require individuals to monitor their own actions and those of others. Whether kids are lock-focused in a competitive game of chess or politely cooperating to build a sandcastle, they must draw on the same executive brain functions, such as being able to evaluate various options, flexibly deal with unexpected developments, and avoid snap judgments that might lead to an unhelpful course of action.

Plus, in both competition and cooperation, a person needs to monitor and anticipate the behavior of the other participant, or predict the other person's moves, which relies heavily on trying to understand the other person's goals and aims in order to more effectively compete or cooperate. The better a child can "read" the other's thoughts, beliefs, desires, and intentions, the more likely they'll be to achieve success in their own goals. Not only that, the more practiced a child is at forming accurate interpretations of what another person is thinking, feeling, and wanting, the more that child can work hard toward a goal while still remaining caring and respectful of others' feelings and differing opinions. That one skill can lead to success not only in competition and cooperation but also in relationships, academics, and nearly every endeavor as they grow up.

> The more skilled a child is at forming accurate interpretations of what another person is thinking, feeling, and wanting, the more that child can work hard toward a goal while still remaining caring and respectful of others' feelings and differing opinions. That one skill can lead to success not only in competition and cooperation but also in relationships, academics, and nearly every endeavor as they grow up.

So what did all this mean for Chloe, and how could her mother, with Georgie's assistance, help her cultivate more empathy at the brain level? One key point they had to keep in mind was that, ironically, this fastidious, determined, single-mindedly-focused-on-winning kid's drive to compete showed that she had *greater* potential, not less, for building additional consideration, compassion, and concern. If Chloe could perform the executive functions necessary to win at competitive games, then she could certainly learn to recruit similar skills to work toward more win-win outcomes that balanced her competitive desires with the feelings of others. Here's how Georgie initially approached Chloe to help nurture her empathy skills, with an unexpected path to getting there—using the nonverbal language of child-led play.

Exercising the Empathy Muscle

Based on what she'd heard, Georgie was a bit surprised by how Chloe entered the office for her first appointment. Rather than confidently striding into the room and announcing her presence, this normally tenacious nine-year-old seemed a little nervous to go into the office. Here's some of what happened when Chloe met Georgie, as the child stood in the doorway:

Chloe: (*Tentatively, a little defensive*) So what am I supposed to do?
Georgie: (*Warmly*) You get to decide what we do here, Chloe. It's up to you.
Chloe: I'm supposed to learn how to play nice.
Georgie: You are?
Chloe: (*Frowning*) But I don't care. And I *don't* want to talk about it.
Georgie: I thought we could just see what you want to do.
Chloe: (*Hopping onto the mini-trampoline, then bouncing*) OK, how (*bounce*) about (*bounce*) this (*bounce, bounce*)?
Georgie: (*Bobbing her head in the same rhythm as Chloe's motions*) You (*bob*) can (*bob*) really (*bob*) jump (*bob, bob*)!
Chloe: Want to jump with me? I mean, there's not enough room on this trampoline, but you can jump right there on the floor.
Georgie: (*Jumping in place, again, matching Chloe's rhythm*) You . . . got it . . . bub!
Chloe: (*Smiling, laughing, still bouncing*) Who you calling bub, *bub*?
Georgie: (*Jumping with each syllable of the singsong phrase*) Who you calling bub, bub!
Chloe: (*In singsong synchrony*) Who you calling bub, bub . . . Who you calling bub, bub . . .
Georgie: (*Continuing to jump with each syllable and chanting the silly, melodic phrase*)
Chloe: (*Suddenly collapsing, giggling*) That was so dumb!
Georgie: But kinda fun?
Chloe: (*Smiling*) It kinda was.

Now that took an unexpected turn! Notice how Georgie responded to the situation. She hadn't at all planned to use the trampoline when Chloe arrived, but she followed her young client's lead and just went with the synchronized silliness. Then soon, almost immediately, the boastful, antagonistic young girl who was supposed to come in looking for competition launched herself into an activity that was friendly and cooperative. That didn't mean, of course, that Chloe would go home a changed person and interact with her family in an entirely new way. But when Georgie spent these few seconds mirroring Chloe's actions (Georgie made herself a mirror), it was the first step toward Chloe sensing a connection with Georgie and allowing it to move into more positive and healthy interactions. Then the next steps could take place, as we'll soon explain.

Many adults think that play is best used as a temporary distraction, something they can grab hold of to divert children's attention away from boredom, difficult feelings, or unruly behavior. We've all seen well-meaning strangers in the grocery store checkout lane, maybe waving a bright-red bag of Doritos in front of a fussy baby in an effort to help a frazzled parent. There's no denying that distraction in these moments can sometimes offer a quick fix.

But play can help us achieve so much more than that. It's one of the most advanced methods we have to practice flexing the empathy muscle—the unique brain structures associated with considering and sensing other people's emotions. And as you're about to see, parents, teachers, therapists, and other adults can use play to encourage children to shift out of negative, unwieldy patterns of behavior that just plain don't work very well for anybody.

> There's no denying that distraction can sometimes offer a quick fix. But play can help us achieve so much more than that. It's one of the most advanced methods we have to practice flexing the empathy muscle—the unique brain structures associated with considering and sensing other people's emotions.

Here's what we've seen so far: (1) Chloe seemed wary of being told she had to change her approach to engaging socially with other people. (2) She also seemed nervous, which appeared out of character for a kid who, by all accounts, usually projected confidence and swagger. And (3) though she felt too defensive to talk about the issues she was having related to others finding her overly competitive, she was willing to open up via a different language that doesn't depend on words. This language is a natural channel of communication kids can access when words fail them: the nonverbal language of play. When kids can't talk about it, they usually can—and do—*play* about it.

> When kids can't talk about it, they usually can—and do—*play* about it.

You can encourage this play-based communication in your kids when you do what Georgie did in this brief interaction with her young client—she made herself a mirror. The basic idea of the strategy is that we mirror what our kids are doing as we play with them. Not copy or mimic them exactly (which would be annoying), but join them in their play, echoing back to them what we see them doing, thereby letting them know that we're attuned to them and to what's important to them. When we do this, all kinds of benefits ensue.

For one thing, the child feels truly *seen*. They probably won't think about it on a conscious level, but by repeatedly joining in what they're doing and clueing in to what they're experiencing and enjoying, we can send the constant message that they matter to us. They also witness, as in the first strategy, that one person can "read" another person's actions and get a sense of what's in their mind.

Empathy proceeds from there. If we can notice when someone else is hurting, we're more likely to *feel with* them, moving beyond mere cognitive empathy to true affective empathy. That means we can better respond with care and sensitivity to our friends, family, and even people who may live differently than we do or who might be socially vulnerable.

> **I**f we can notice when someone else is hurting, we're more likely to *feel with* them, moving beyond mere cognitive empathy to true affective empathy. That means we can better respond with care and sensitivity to our friends, family, and even people who may live differently than we do or who might be socially vulnerable.

It follows, then, that if we can pay attention to the minds of others, we can observe and be more aware of what's happening in our own minds. In fact, the acts of seeing our own minds and seeing the minds of others are intimately tied to each other, as the prefrontal cortex gives rise to both of these functions.

They are so closely connected that two prominent researchers in our field have coined terms that bring the concepts together. Dan Siegel created the term "mindsight," which is essentially the ability to see and understand our own minds as well as the minds of others. Think of it as a combo of insight and empathy. Peter Fonagy's term "mentalization" is similar. He describes it as the ability to see thoughts, feelings, intentions, and the internal experiences beneath the external behaviors of ourselves and others, or "having one's mind in mind."

Both researchers have written extensively about these complex processes, and we're giving only a simple explanation here, but know that this notion is more revolutionary than it might appear. Too often, kids (and adults) simply react to situations without considering what they're feeling or how they'd actually like to behave. But if they can observe their own minds, as well as others' minds, and notice that they are, say, angry or afraid or something else, then they will be much more apt to actually *decide* how they will respond to what's before them rather than just unconsciously reacting. What this means, practically, is that anytime we help kids tune in to their own minds, or anytime we help them attune to other minds, we're helping them flex and strengthen their brains' ability with *both* functions.

We performed a thought experiment in the previous chapter where we asked you to consider how your family life might change if your child developed some of the skills we're discussing. Let's ask that question again here. Just think about the impact it could have on the dynamics in your home if your child were more empathetic and better able to see within their own mind—even to a small extent—before simply reacting when faced with a difficult or emotional situation. Imagine, too, how valuable these skills will be as your child grows into a teenager, then an adult. Then consider the difference when they become a parent. The abilities that can result from your mirroring and the other strategies we'll be discussing can have truly generational effects.

> Just think about the impact it could have on the family dynamics in your home if your child were more empathetic and better able to see within their own mind— even to a small extent—before simply reacting when faced with a difficult or emotional situation.

Are we saying that all of this will happen overnight, or from one session on the trampoline? Of course not. But over time, when your kids receive daily reminders that they matter to you—that you'll give them your time, that you'll consistently spend a few minutes engaging with them in an activity they love—they will receive a powerful message that they matter, not only to you but as participants in this world.

And over the next few years, as they spend more time away from you at school and with friends and then eventually leave home, they'll do so from a place of confidence and independence that's been created and fostered by the time they've spent with you. They'll approach their worlds with a deeper understanding of their emotional lives and what that means in their interactions with others.

That's why we say it's a mindset that you want to create within yourself. Yes, we're showing you simple and practical ways you can use playtime to help your kids develop optimally, but the key to the whole PlayStrong approach is that it becomes a way of *being* with your children, where all the various strategies work together and lay a relational foundation that allows your children to live into the fullness of who they can be.

> Yes, we're showing you simple and practical ways you can use playtime to help your kids develop optimally, but the key to the whole PlayStrong approach is that it becomes a way of *being* with your children, where all the various strategies work together and lay a relational foundation that allows your children to live into the fullness of who they can be.

The Power of "Bottom Up"

One of the most exciting discoveries in the world of neuroscience over the last few decades has to do with mirror neurons. The discovery occurred in 1992 when a team of Italian researchers stumbled upon a subset of neural cells that fired whenever a macaque monkey picked up or ate a bit of peanut or banana, *and* when the monkey merely watched another monkey or human do the same thing.

At first it didn't make any sense—the activated brain cells were supposed to be motor neurons, the kind that should fire only when the monkey lifted its hand to grasp and eat its own peanut. But soon the scientists realized that these special clusters of neurons in the premotor cortex were also capable of sensing and detecting a motor action in *another* monkey or human, from merely watching others move their hand to pick up a peanut. "You know what that feels like, too!" the neurons seemed to be saying. The Italian team dubbed their unexpected discovery "mirror neurons" and pointed to the strong possibility that they are part of a mapping system that exists in the brain that helps us recognize and relate to others' actions.

Do the findings apply to humans? Many researchers feel confident that they do, as subsequent studies have identified a similar mirroring system in the human brain. While there's still much we don't know about the subject, and implications for what mirror neurons explain are still being debated, this discovery is a significant contribution in helping scientists explain how we "read" other people's minds and feel empathy for them.

Looking back at the way Chloe played with Georgie—and specifically what she chose to do when there weren't any perceived expectations and she wasn't pressuring herself to perform—we see that this nine-year-old girl began to seek Georgie's attention in a remarkable way. As Chloe bounced up and down on the trampoline, she offered Georgie—a brand-new adult she had met only moments earlier—the opportunity to mirror her actions. As she bounced, she created a rhythm in the timing of her jumps, the melodic cadence of her voice, and the repetition in her speech ("Who you calling *bub*, bub") that another person could easily match. It's as if she *craved* to be mirrored.

That's what Georgie offered when she made herself a mirror. In bouncing with her and repeating with her the singsong phrase, she was actually communicating with Chloe's brain and nervous system. There wasn't a conscious process or thought at work as they jumped, but something was happening deep down below the higher, more conscious parts of the brain. This type of mirroring is what we call a "bottom-up process."

Different from a top-down approach, bottom-up processing has much less to do with thinking, or with logical or verbal explanations. Instead, it relies primarily on the senses, and it carries messages up to the brain from the body. Examples of bottom-up processing are when you hear a noise and immediately turn your head, or when you jerk your hand back from a hot stove. Your senses are sending signals that your higher brain hasn't even processed yet. Those signals are sent from the bottom up—or as pediatric psychologist Mona Delahooke puts it, "body up."

Top-down processing, on the other hand, relies mainly on the "top" or higher structures of the brain, such as the prefrontal cortex. These upper parts of the brain do the higher-order thinking—they problem-solve, process words, address problems, and much more. So "top down" means using the top of our nervous system, specifically the cortex, which is the higher parts of the brain in our skull.

When Georgie imitated Chloe, the young girl's body gathered and sent information upward to the lower parts of her brain, and then on up to the cortex, where her mirror neurons could "read" what it meant. It was a bottom-up process. Again, Chloe wouldn't have actually thought, "This therapist and I are resonating in some way," but something beneath her consciousness, in her body, got the message. That might not mean that much in a one-time interaction, but when that kind of relational joining occurs again and again, as it did in subsequent interactions with Georgie, it becomes extraordinarily powerful. The trampoline mirroring, in other words, was the beginning of a relationship between Chloe and Georgie, and it created a foundation they would build on in the coming weeks.

Along the way, Georgie used more top-down strategies with Chloe as well, and she taught the concepts to Annie, who before long began reporting back that the simple act of mirroring changed everything. Chloe seemed to be more aware of, and interested in, the inner workings of others. She kept playing at home with her mom. She still struggled with being overly competitive on a regular basis—that was part of her personality and what made her tick, after all—but over time, the whole family could tell they were making progress and enjoying one another's company much more.

TOP-DOWN PROCESSING USES WORDS AND LOGIC
TO SEND SIGNALS FROM HIGHER PARTS OF THE BRAIN
DOWN TO THE BODY.

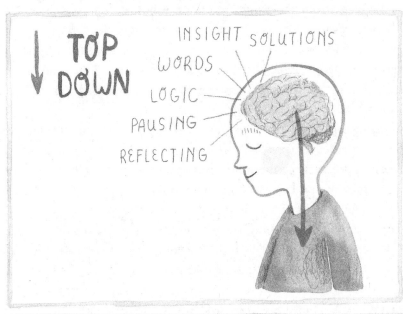

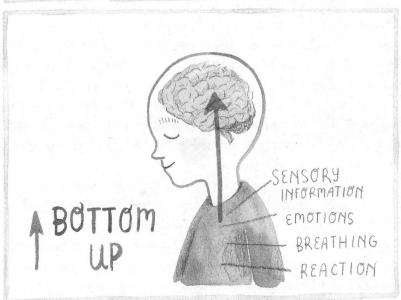

BOTTOM-UP PROCESSING RELIES PRIMARILY ON THE SENSES,
THE BODY, AND LOWER STRUCTURES OF THE BRAIN,
CARRYING MESSAGES UP TO THE HIGHER PARTS
OF THE BRAIN FROM THE BODY.

Making yourself a mirror is a natural precursor to establishing a warm and genuine connection in developing relationships at every stage. Not only does it help us figure out how others are feeling, but the experience of being mirrored makes us instantly feel seen, understood, and valued. Thanks to our mirror neurons, our minds can understand those around us. It's similar to the process described in studies that found that when researchers imitated subjects' body posture (e.g., leaning forward, crossing legs), the subjects were much more likely to show kindness to the researcher, a complete stranger, and pick up a set of pens that the researcher intentionally spilled on the ground. The subjects couldn't explain why, but they wanted to be more caring and helpful toward the stranger who mirrored them, showing appreciation in immediate and practical ways.

> Not only does mirroring help us figure out how others are feeling, but the experience of being mirrored makes us instantly feel seen, understood, and valued.

It's been shown that mirroring others can lead to more intimacy, trust, cooperation, positive emotion, and emotional understanding. This is true for all kinds of dyads—romantic partners, teachers and students, bosses and employees, parents and kids, and more.

As parents, we can tap into the power of mirroring whenever we need to give kids a boost of connection that will shift their moods and attitudes toward the positive. If you want to feel closer to your child, and you want them to feel more optimistic and cooperative toward you and others, making yourself a mirror is one of the quickest ways to get there. Some of you might already know this. What we're discussing might already be a part of your parenting repertoire. For others, this approach may feel revolutionary. Our hope is that regardless of how intuitive the following steps may (or may not) feel, you'll get a clear sense of how powerful it can be to connect with your child simply by mirroring their actions.

Make Yourself a Mirror: Step by Step

When you and your child begin to play, don't put pressure on yourself to know exactly what to do. Just engage with their open-ended ideas in their current activity, looking for opportunities to switch on mirror neurons—first yours, then theirs—using the old "monkey see, monkey do" technique.

Step 1: Observe and attune, using your own mirror neurons

Just as you did in the first PlayStrong strategy, start here by simply observing and attuning to your child as they play. Watch what they're doing and identify some action you can imitate nonverbally. Just pay attention and see what you notice.

For example, imagine a mom—let's call her Madeline—who's in the backyard pitching a Wiffle ball to her baseball-crazy son. He

USE YOUR OWN MIRROR NEURONS.

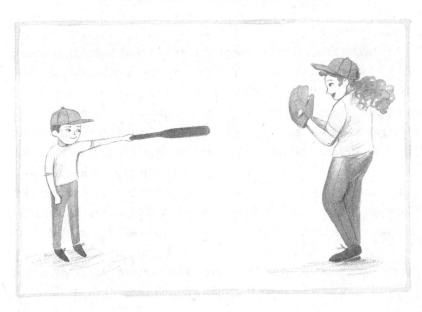

grabs his bat and steps up to the plate, then points the bat right at Madeline, the pitcher, just as he saw his favorite player do during last night's game. Her first job is simply to notice this move and the details involved: the grave look on his face, his squinting eyes, the way he subtly nods his head toward her.

Step 2: Activate your child's mirror system
Once Madeline has noticed these particular details, she then mirrors them back to her son, letting him know, without ever saying anything, that she's clued in and connected to his presence. She points back at him, the same stern look on her face, with a slight nod. Mother and son are in sync.

ACTIVATE YOUR CHILD'S MIRROR SYSTEM.

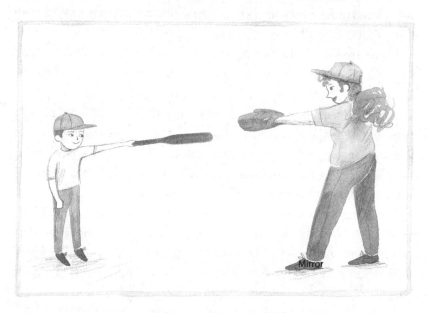

That's it—that's the whole thing! We're serious. That interaction between parent and child is worth more than most people ever know, in terms of the child's optimal development and the relationship he enjoys with his mom.

Why? What's going on in this moment, and why is it so powerful? Well, for one thing, the oldest evolutionary pathways in the brain are nonverbal. Your actions always speak louder than words when it comes to your child's mind.

> The oldest evolutionary pathways in the brain are nonverbal. Your actions practically always speak louder than words when it comes to your child's mind.

So what's happening here is that the son is understanding, at a deep, unconscious level, that his mother is completely attuned, immersed in the moment the two are sharing. Down below the surface of awareness, this boy is registering that his mom is in sync with him. That she gets him.

Compare this interaction to one where our child plays near us and says, "Look, Mom!" and we briefly look up from our phone and offer a distracted "That's nice, honey." We've all done it, and a less-than-attentive response isn't going to ruin our kids. Plus, the kind of concentrated, engaged play we're talking about here is something that you'd do only at certain points each day. In other words, you wouldn't have Madeline's focus every second with your child. That would be impossible, not to mention unhealthy for both of you.

We bring up the uninterested response from the mom simply to contrast it with the focused mirroring during Madeline's moment playing with her son to highlight the difference in a child's experience when they receive that kind of attention and mirroring from a parent.

Notice that Madeline isn't doing anything complicated here. She's simply mirroring what she sees. To be more specific, she's employing what we call the BFVs: body, face, and voice.

For one thing, she mirrored her son's body by picking out the pointing gesture. There's no right decision here; she simply chose this gesture since that worked in her situation. When you use it with your kids, you'll mirror with your own body based on the circumstances

MIRROR YOUR CHILD USING THE BFVS.

B: *With your BODY*

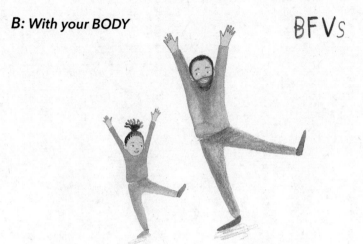

BFVs

F: *With your FACE*

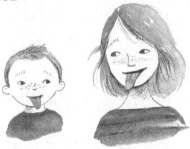

V: *With your VOICE*

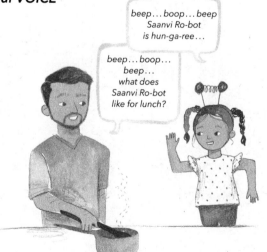

MIRROR WITH YOUR BODY.

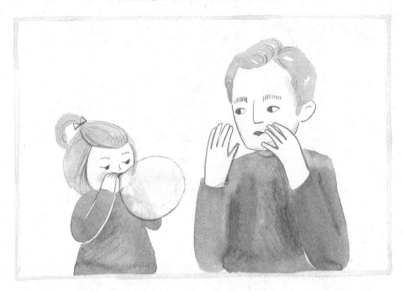

of your situation. You might, for example, focus on a physical movement, like tapping a toe; or a gesture, such as taking a bow; or body posture, like sitting up straight or leaning forward or lounging on the floor. The point is simply to mirror what you see your child doing with their body.

MIRROR WITH YOUR BODY.

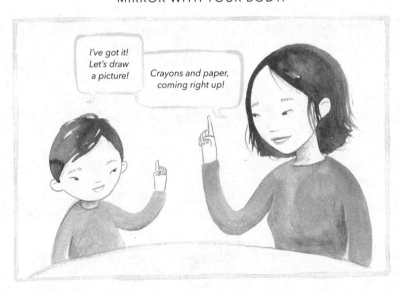

MIRROR WITH YOUR FACE.

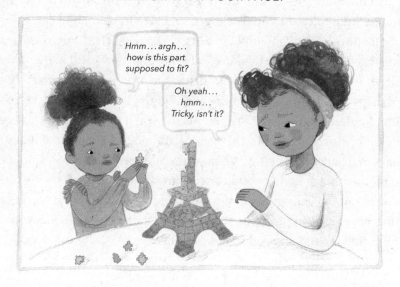

You can also mirror with your face, matching your child's expressions with your own. Imagine, for example, that your daughter is struggling with a difficult puzzle, her eyebrows furrowed as she concentrates to solve it. When she looks up and sees that you're reflecting something similar with your facial expressions in that moment, she'll get the sense that you see, you understand, and you care.

MIRROR WITH YOUR FACE.

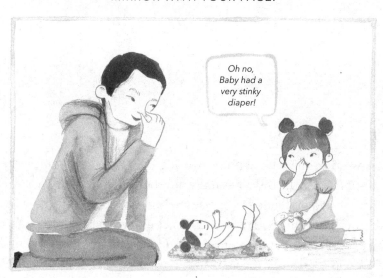

So those are the "B" and the "F" of BFV. The third main mirroring tool is your voice. As you play together, listen to your child and think about how you might imitate certain vocal or rhythmic qualities. Maybe you notice a particular vocal tone, high and shrill like a police siren, low and deep like a bass drum, or anything in between. Or perhaps you'll notice something about your child's volume, like getting louder or quiet as a whisper. Maybe you'll create rhyme or keep in time with your child's rhythm, or add sound effects like a dog's bark or a helicopter flying. When your child uses their voice, your job is simply to echo what you hear to show how it resonates with you. You're not typically going to just ricochet back exactly what you hear. Instead, engage in the moment in a way that demonstrates that you're fully clued in to what your child is doing.

MIRROR WITH YOUR VOICE.

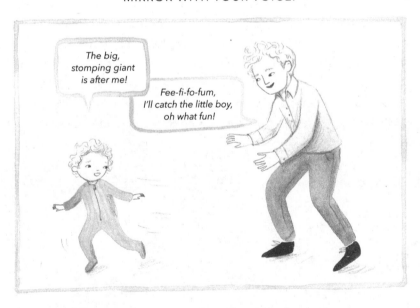

A word to the wise about mirroring: You may have noticed here that sometimes the BFVs naturally dovetail with one another, such as when the dad pretended to be a stomping giant: (1) doing the stomping steps (with his body), and (2) voicing the deeper tone (with his voice) of the giant at the same time. Often, as in this case, two of the BFVs will work well together. But beware of using all three BFVs simultaneously. It's common knowledge that people of all ages detest being copied exactly word-for-word, or action-by-action. In fact, being a copycat is one of the main tactics kids deploy to annoy one another! So in order to be more successful with your nonverbal BFVs, try not to use all three—body, face, and voice—at once.

MIRROR WITH YOUR VOICE.

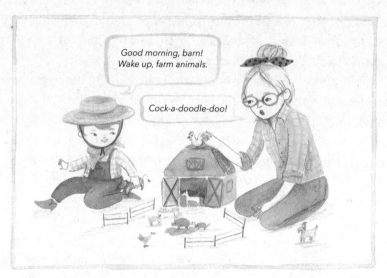

And if you can help it, avoid repeating what children say verbatim. Imitation may be the sincerest form of flattery, but it loses originality if someone is robotically repeating your words back to you. With subtle gestures and good timing, though, kids love being mirrored, especially if your movements, expressions, and sounds add authentic feeling or expand on what's going on during playtime.

> With subtle gestures and good timing, kids love being mirrored, especially if your movements, expressions, and sounds add authentic feeling or expand on what's going on during playtime.

One other warning: As with virtually any other interaction with your kids, it's important to keep in mind the developmental stage of your child while using this strategy. What creates glee for a three-year-old—big facial expressions and a singsong voice—might be a huge turnoff to a nine-year-old. And what's more, two different three-year-olds may have very different responses to the same mirroring you offer. So when you play, make a point to concentrate on providing what *this particular child* needs and enjoys. This isn't a one-size-fits-all kind of endeavor. (That's why the first step, once again, is to observe *and attune*.)

The simplicity of what we're teaching here might make you wonder whether mirroring can be as powerful as we're saying. But give it a shot, putting it to use alongside the other strategies from the book, and see what you discover. The truth is, our kids just want us to connect with them. It's the connected parent, the one who knows how to mirror what their child is feeling deep inside, who can help heal the hurts and make their child feel whole. By taking a few minutes to reflect your child's simple but important signals, you can assist them toward developing valuable life skills that come with increased empathy and social intelligence. They'll be better able to understand themself; identify what others feel just by listening to and looking at them; show more empathy and kindness as they personally relate to others' experiences; and respond with more care and sensitivity to their friends, family, and even people they have conflict with.

Making ourselves a mirror flips the empathy switch in our children, releasing a cascade of brain-based social skills and abilities, allowing your child to tap into more emotionally connected behaviors that will bring others closer and deepen their ability to socialize with nuanced and heartfelt reflection.

Notice, too, the way these skills create a scaffolding effect with those produced by the first PlayStrong strategy. The main focus there is on helping kids become aware of, understand, and express their inner worlds. Much of this second strategy will generate similar effects in your kids, while also helping them take that self-understanding and expand it into more meaningful awareness of and connection to the people around them. Now, in the next strategy, we'll show you how you can develop these capabilities and help your kids be aware of the inner worlds of themselves and others, and use that awareness to regulate their own actions and treat others in kinder and more respectful ways.

Bring Emotions to Life

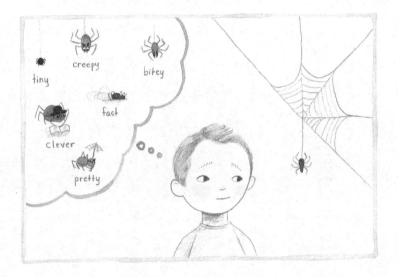

Primary skill being developed in the child:
The ability to recognize, manage, and express emotions.

Primary message received by the child:
Someone will help me recognize and make sense of my big feelings.

By this point you've learned two simple strategies—Think Out Loud and Make Yourself a Mirror—that you can use to help build skills like self-awareness and empathy within your child. Now let's turn to feelings—specifically, helping your kids develop the ability to regulate their own emotions and handle themselves well, even when they face really difficult situations.

Sometimes children need assistance on the most basic level of recognizing their own feelings and what they mean; sometimes they need help managing them once they recognize them; and sometimes they need help expressing and releasing their emotions when those feelings threaten to overwhelm them.

Our third PlayStrong strategy, Bring Emotions to Life, focuses on all three of these needs: helping kids recognize, manage, and express their feelings. By leaning in to emotions expressed in play, you can help your child practice emotional regulation and let go of big feelings that are not helping them, thus reducing the chaotic behavior and reactivity that so often comes with pent-up emotion.

Children and Emotions

A toddler cries at daycare drop-off. A second grader's best friend moves away. A fourth grader worries about doing well in school and fitting in with peers. When children experience scary, sad, stressful, disappointing, or painful moments, it can be overwhelming (for kids and parents alike).

And those challenges appear from the very beginning. Toddlers most certainly discover that they have big feelings when they want to go down the slide but everyone must wait their turn. Ideally, they begin to understand that there are different ways people express basic feelings, and they learn to let people know when they feel happy, sad, mad, excited, afraid. They learn how to tune in to their bodies so they can recognize their feelings and express them in acceptable ways. And the most profound emotional and relational learning—the kind that develops a child's ability to weather emotional storms—comes from the most basic interactions kids share with their parents and families, as well as their teachers and friends, all the way through childhood and adolescence.

> The most profound emotional and relational learning—the kind that develops a child's ability to weather emotional storms—comes from the most basic interactions kids share with their parents and families, as well as their teachers and friends, all the way through childhood and adolescence.

At every point along their journey, we can help children "bring emotions to life," thus transforming their difficult feelings into manageable, meaningful experiences that build their brains and deepen our relationship with them.

The Emotional Brain

An enormous percentage of everything we and our kids do is intimately tied to our emotions. And a huge portion of what we feel, and therefore how we behave, depends on the *context* of what's happening in a given situation. That environmental context—what's going on inside ourselves as well as what we see, hear, and experience in relation to those around us—largely determines our feelings and how we emotionally encode and regulate these important moments. That's why we want to bring emotions to life.

It's helpful to know just a bit about what happens in the brain when we interact with and encode these experiences. As you know, the brain is very complex, and there's still plenty to learn about the workings of the nervous system, of which the brain is a part. So we need to be careful when making claims about which parts of the brain handle which bodily processes. That said, there are parts of the brain that do specialize, in coordination with other parts, in processing, appraising, and regulating emotions and stress.

One of these instrumental areas has been traditionally called the limbic system or limbic region. Made up of the amygdala and hippocampus, in coordination with the rest of the nervous system, it contains one of the essential brain mechanisms that gives rise to happiness, fear, anger, shame, sadness, and our other complex emotions. These various feelings are key to helping the brain make meaning out of assorted sensations—messages that travel via electrochemical signals from the body through the nervous system and brainstem, right up to the limbic structures of the brain's middle layer. Sometimes called the emotional nervous system, the limbic area collects any information the body can share about what we're feeling, then it comes up with a corresponding emotion, an outward expression of the most accurate label it can find for the feelings we're experiencing internally.

When you walk through a beautiful garden, enjoying the sensory input of sights and smells all around you, the limbic region contributes to giving you the warm, tranquil feeling that you experience as happiness or pleasure. Likewise, if a bee in that garden drifts over and lands on your hand, then the whole context suddenly changes. Prepared to respond to even the slightest hint of danger, the limbic area and its substructures, such as the amygdala, hypothalamus, and hippocampus, become alert to the offending bee and its tiny stinger hovering above your skin. Unless you adore bees and are not afraid, these structures may send a cascade of fight-or-flight signals to your body, causing fear sensations and reflexive body movements so you can flick your hand away and swiftly evade a painful sting. You can thank your limbic region, as well as the brainstem's faster-than-lightning signal carrying, for getting you out of harm's way in the nick of time. Just as the serene environment originally created positive emotions within you, the threat of being stung produces fear and the appropriate response to that potential reality.

The point is that those emotions are constantly swirling around within us based on what we experience in our moment-to-moment circumstances. They can crop up before we have a chance to think them through or even notice them in the lightning-fast, bottom-up processing that the lower structures of our brains perform to protect us. Sometimes that's a good thing, like in the bee example. But when it comes to relationships, we'd like to be a bit more intentional with our responses. We therefore need to develop the capacity to notice those feelings so we can make decisions about how best to respond to them, rather than unconsciously reacting to what we're feeling without even considering whether that reaction is appropriate or helpful in a given situation. Our kids need to develop the same set of abilities—they need to learn to bring emotions to life.

The limbic part of our brain plays a key role in this process. It helps make sense of the multitude of sensations and impulses we're experiencing millisecond by millisecond. For example, imagine that you're with your son as he examines and admires a spiderweb, reveling in the intricacies of the spider's handiwork. Then, suddenly, he sees the actual spider attached to the web. At this point he might feel apprehensive as he works through the assorted associations he might have about spiders.

THE BRAIN IS AN ASSOCIATION MACHINE THAT CAN OFFER DIFFERENT INTERPRETATIONS OF OUR CIRCUMSTANCES.

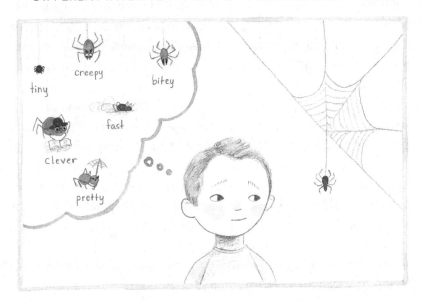

In this moment of limbic appraisal, which interpretation of the spider will win out? How will your son end up feeling? A split second is all it takes to work through this complicated, often-unconscious process and fit the spider into its current context.

THE BRAIN IS AN ASSOCIATION MACHINE THAT CAN OFFER DIFFERENT INTERPRETATIONS OF OUR CIRCUMSTANCES.

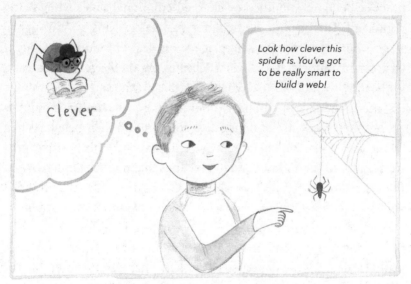

Every time a child faces a situation that asks them to process their emotions, it's an opportunity to build skills in that area. And as you might imagine, play is one of the best ways to repeatedly give them that opportunity. Just as your child would spend many hours rehearsing before a piano recital or practicing with their soccer team before the next big game, dramatic play muscles up the limbic region with a huge variety of "trying on" emotions and situations in preparation for dealing with emotions more effectively in real time. As the research increasingly shows, play is one of the most important vehicles we have for assisting the next generation to practice emotional-intelligence abilities such as self-control, pausing, and using social skills in a risk-free environment.

By strategically joining your child in a dramatic play scenario and helping them bring their emotions to life, you give them the chance to "play through" their feelings—to name, experience, and discuss their emotions calmly and explicitly, when they're not in the heat of the moment, unwilling or unable to think clearly or even talk about what's going on inside themselves.

Put differently, play helps children learn to manage their biggest, scariest, and most difficult feelings without having an actual fight-flight-freeze stress response. In fact, play *reduces* stress, so they get practice being in amplified or charged emotional states while being regulated! This is foundational for resilience. Kids go through a stage where they need a safe place to project emotions that might be too uncomfortable or overwhelming for their age. In this case, it's healthy for kids to use what experts call "the safety of symbolic distance." There, they can have different characters, dolls, or puppets act out their most stressful, negative emotions on their behalf. When emotions are just too big to manage, children need this positive, projective play to see and understand feelings that might be much bigger than they are. When it's "not about me," children can safely interact with their own feelings and develop a sense of mastery over them.

You can help your child bring these emotions to life by playfully acting them out on their behalf. This shows that these emotions, though they might make people feel frightened or vulnerable for a short time, can be managed effectively. In other words, we can survive difficult feelings by projecting them in play so they can be reintegrated within the safety of symbolic play.

Bear in mind that our emotions are going to be at work within us whether we pay attention to them or not. That's where the real danger—as well as the real possibility—lies. There's nothing at all wrong with feeling angry; that's an important and even healthy part of the whole range of human emotion and the human experience. But when we're mad and *we don't know* that we're mad, and we can't regulate the intensity of it, we can act in ways that get us into trouble, ways that can even become destructive. The same goes for fear, anxiety, depression, and other powerful emotions. We need to bring them into the light of awareness—to bring them to life—because they'll be influencing us whether we realize we're experiencing them or not.

So a principle that underpins this third strategy, and really the entire PlayStrong approach, is that we need to allow and even encourage kids to experience their emotions in a safe environment, and use that limbic experience to help them better understand their big feelings. When we give them repeated practice at feeling and interacting with emotions, they'll be able to handle their emotions more effectively and appropriately in other areas of their lives. Kids learn about their emotions by getting to actually experience them and then work through them.

> Kids learn about their emotions by getting to actually experience them and then work through them.

Play Lays the Foundation for Emotional Regulation and Better Decision-Making

Play is one of the most powerful ways to help our kids develop as optimally as possible. In this case, it offers a safe environment for them to practice feeling their emotions so they can handle themselves better in intense situations. Here's how the process works.

First, through play, we give children the opportunity to safely experience virtually all of their emotions. Then, we teach them to notice and become aware of those feelings. This limbic-to-cortex linkage process begins when children are extremely young and continues well into adolescence and even young adulthood. The very act of noticing what we're feeling is a powerful skill that all of us need in order to succeed in life.

That recognition, then, leads to kids' ability to *name* their feelings once they've noticed them. In doing so they'll be able to more effectively regulate those emotions. Then that leads to one of the key goals of the process, helping them not only notice and name their emotions but also express them in appropriate ways and make better decisions. Kids (like adults) won't be perfect at doing so, but even at young ages they really can improve at noticing, naming, regulating, and expressing their emotions in appropriate ways. From there, we can help build more and stronger emotional and relational skills so that they're less likely to become overwhelmed when they're faced with demanding and difficult circumstances. This is what "bringing emotions to life" is all about.

PLAY HELPS KIDS MOVE FROM EXPERIENCING EMOTIONS TO MAKING BETTER DECISIONS.

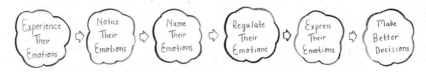

We hope this comes as hopeful news for parents, teachers, therapists, and other caring adults actively looking for ways to support kids around emotions. Play really can reduce emotional reactivity and teach children to lean in to difficult feelings rather than react to them. This is one of the reasons we called this book *The Way of Play*! This is the way we can give our kids repeated positive experiences associated with understanding their emotional lives and then regulating and expressing their feelings.

Then, as they mature, they can develop healthy emotional lives rather than developing patterns of running from feelings, distracting themselves, numbing out, or reacting without choice. We want to make sure parents understand this one key piece of information that's absolutely fundamental to the way we approach our children's emotions, no matter how straightforward or challenging they may be: If you want your child to learn how to manage their emotions, you've first got to let the emotions live and breathe. You've got to bring them to life.

> If you want your child to learn how to manage their emotions, you've first got to let the emotions live and breathe. You've got to bring them to life.

We can divide emotion-based play into three main types, based on the limbic benefits offered by each: expressive play, preventative play, and responsive play.

Emotion-Based Play Type #1: Expressive Play

Expressive play is likely the type of emotion-based play you're most familiar with. It involves helping children develop what experts call an "emotional vocabulary," so they can more fully notice and recognize the feelings within themselves. Key to this strategy is watching for play situations that create drama and allowing children to pay attention to and begin to name the emotions that spring up along the way. When you play with them the game where they avoid the "lava" that your living room rug has become, you are really talking about the emotion of fear. Not in a forced "Let's discuss what we're feeling" kind of way, but naturally, as part of the game.

And when the playacting later turns to anxiety about whether the wicked queen has cast a spell on the apple, you can name the nervousness that the characters would be feeling.

USE PLAYTIME TO HELP TEACH ABOUT FEELINGS.

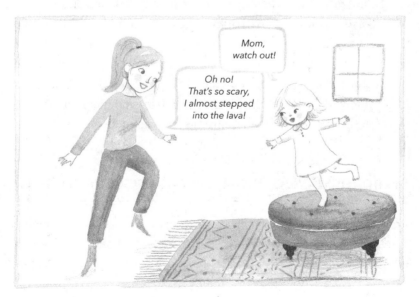

USE PLAYTIME TO HELP TEACH ABOUT FEELINGS.

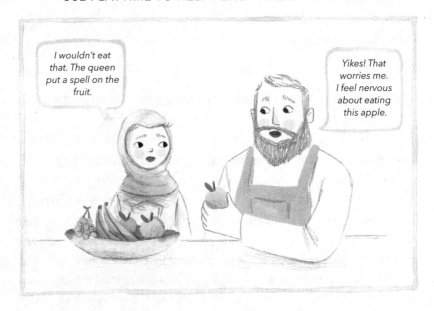

As is so often the case when we discuss the power of play, there's nothing mysterious or magical going on here (other than the spell on the fruit!), and you don't have to be a child-development expert to participate. These two respective parents are simply naming emotions, giving their kids the opportunity to learn the words for various emotions and to connect them to their play-based fantasies.

As they grow up and face frightening and challenging situations in the real world, they'll be much better equipped to deal with authentic fear and actual anxiety because they have a hardy and robust emotional vocabulary that you've helped them develop during playtime. Plus, you will have given them repeated experiences of working through those emotions, where things worked out in the end.

Emotion-Based Play Type #2: Preventative Play

Preventative play does just what you'd expect based on its name: It helps prevent future problems and behavioral issues through the medium of play. When children physically engage in dramatic play, they're really pretending to experience the emotions, behaviors, and mental states of other people, and in the safety of "just pretend," they experience new situations that might ordinarily feel too foreign or frightening to engage with in the real world.

Social psychologist Thalia Goldstein has led pioneering studies on the positive effects of children acting out emotions in dramatic play and role-taking. Goldstein discovered that kids who spend more time in dramatic play—thinking about how people interact and assigning meaning to behaviors and emotional states—score significantly higher on measures of emotional and relational intelligence. Compared to children assigned randomly to groups building with blocks or listening to a story, kids who engaged in short sessions of guided pretend play with teachers—where they were asked to explore characters' motivations and embody the feelings of different personalities—showed (forgive the pun) dramatic improvements in emotional self-control and positive social behaviors. What's more, playing pretend didn't just improve kids' self-control in the moment. The positive behavioral changes "generalized," which means they actually held up in other moments, between acting sessions and even after the study was concluded!

> Kids who spend more time in dramatic play—thinking about how people interact and assigning meaning to behaviors and emotional states—score significantly higher on measures of emotional and relational intelligence.

So what was special about the children who were invited to frolic around the room like jungle animals or whip up pretend meals for classmates like a chef? These dramatic games stimulated a limbic workout unlike any other, training the kids' emotional-management systems to engage in a wider variety of feelings, trying on different emotions and providing plenty of repeated opportunities to practice handling complex emotions in a simulated environment. Letting kids work through emotional drama in play, when "it's not real, only pretend," creates the potential for a stronger limbic capacity—which means these kids will be more prepared to take charge of real emotions when they arise. It can actually prevent future problems.

And while toys are great, when kids use their own bodies in the place of dolls or action figures, we are more likely to see their emotions come to life, resulting in these marked increases in emotional self-control in line with Dr. Goldstein's findings. Why? Because when kids safely explore emotions, both mentally *and* physically, role-playing with their whole bodies, they develop a stronger limbic brain-body connection. Learning cognitive skills, such as pointing to happy or sad faces on a printable chart, is an excellent way to teach children explicit basic knowledge of emotions, but it appeals primarily to higher levels of the brain that are better at processing information when kids are calm. It's a top-down process.

On the other hand, when they act out real-life scenarios, their bodies are suddenly bombarded with more intense or complex emotions—like feeling enraged, panicky, isolated, baffled, or jealous. Adding in this bottom-up process allows children to gain more from this type of playacting that focuses *also* on emotions versus more top-down cognitive skills alone. The reason is that this feeling-plus-thinking activity integrates many of the differentiated, yet interconnected, parts of the brain, body, and nervous system.

Obviously, it's not that we expect our kids to grow up to be firefighters or interstellar pioneers—at least, not necessarily. But with each opportunity they receive to experience heightened emotions during play, they'll more fully develop their ability to handle stressful situations they face away from home. In other words, they'll learn to navigate an emotionally complex world. They can learn about controlling anger by becoming a charging elephant who also chooses to stop before damaging a family's car, just as they can strengthen their sense of responsibility by taking on the role of a superhero, having mere seconds to save an entire city from a crushing tidal wave.

PRETEND PLAY HELPS KIDS DEAL WITH BIG EMOTIONS IN SAFE
SITUATIONS SO THEY CAN BETTER HANDLE REAL-WORLD
CHALLENGES WHEN THEY COME.

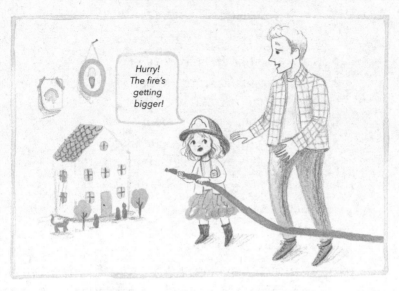

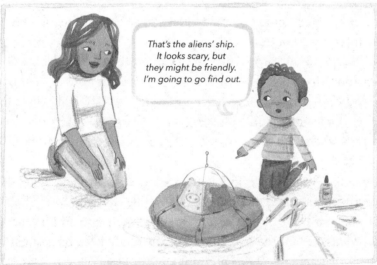

If you want your child to get lots of repetition dealing with emotionally charged situations, and your goal is to fortify their ability to
manage their own feelings with more ease and confidence, playing
proactively to build emotional skills is one of the best ways to get
there. Then, once children have already acquired better skills, they'll

be primed ahead of time to process emotions more competently when real-world challenges come their way.

> If you want your child to get lots of repetition dealing with emotionally charged situations, and your goal is to fortify their ability to manage their own feelings with more ease and confidence, playing proactively to build emotional skills is one of the best ways to get there.

Emotion-Based Play Type #3: Responsive Play

Our final type of emotion-based play has to do with using pretend play to express emotions and release them so they don't come out in less-than-optimal ways. After all, it's often the case that kids don't even know that they're experiencing powerful emotions in their bodies, and/or they're unable to talk about what they're feeling. So in that situation, play offers this other emotional language that parents can tap into when kids can't express their emotions in words. As we've said before, when kids can't *say* it, they can often *play* it.

Imagine, for example, that you have a five-year-old daughter who recently had a scary choking incident while eating grapes. She was safe afterward, but it becomes clear that the frightening event has stayed with her for the next few days. She might keep bringing it up, or begin eating only yogurt and soup, refusing solid foods. Once you notice these new signs that she's having trouble moving past the experience, it would seem pretty clear that the fear and panic from the moment are very much still working on her. Even if she isn't aware that those emotions are active in her mind and body, they definitely are.

WHEN KIDS CAN'T SAY IT, THEY OFTEN PLAY IT.

One of the best ways you could help her, then, would be to provide her with an opportunity to reframe that experience when you play with her. You might set up a table with a tray of pretend food and invite her teddy bear to join the two of you. During the pretend meal, then, you might notice that she is warning her teddy not to eat too fast since "it might get stuck." You could highlight her efforts to feed the bear slowly, encouraging him to take small bites and chew thoroughly, assuring Teddy that he'll be safe, that he's eaten solid foods ever since he was tiny. And you could do the same while taking pretend bites of play food yourself.

With further interactions like this, your daughter can feel more in control of her fear that's bound to get expressed in her body while she plays, and she can feel more confident in solving the problem in your safe presence.

Notice that this becomes possible when your daughter has you there, involved in her playtime. Don't get us wrong: Kids can, and do, work through emotional dilemmas when they play with peers and when they play alone. Indeed, children need lots of free, open-ended, independent play to experience all the benefits we're discussing in this book. But another active ingredient to improving your child's

RESPONSIVE PLAY HELPS KIDS EXPRESS EMOTIONS AND THEN RELEASE THEM SO THEY DON'T COME OUT IN LESS-THAN-OPTIMAL WAYS.

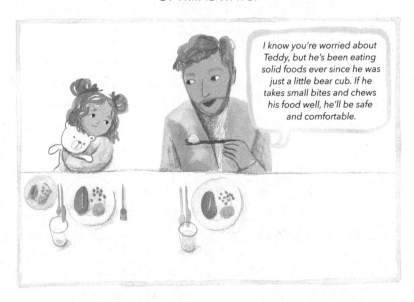

emotional intelligence is you being there, offering a few minutes each day to bring in the right strategy and get those limbic brain-body connections going in the context of their safe relationship with you.

> Another active ingredient to improving your child's emotional intelligence is you being there, offering a few minutes each day to bring in the right strategy and get those limbic brain-body connections going in the context of their safe relationship with you.

Bring Emotions to Life: Step by Step

You've seen several examples already of how you can use your play-time with your kids to bring their emotions to life and help them develop into children, then later teens and adults, with healthy and dynamic social and emotional intelligence and agility. Now let's get a bit more specific about the practical steps for bringing emotions to life. Here's how you can approach play as a limbic-to-cortex exercise, broadening your child's vocabulary of feelings and strengthening the emotionally intelligent, meaning-making connections between your child's body and brain.

Step 1: Observe and attune, watching for emotional cues

As with the other PlayStrong strategies, Bring Emotions to Life begins by having you simply tune in to your kid and observe what's taking place in their mind. You're joining with your child in their play, but you're allowing them to take the lead. Especially for this third strategy— which uses dramatic play to help foreground emotional issues in your interactions with your child—your job is to notice where they're going, then ride along beside them, nudging the process at times but allowing them to remain in control of where things are headed. A helpful analogy is to think of your child as a movie director who's creating characters and determining the plot of the dramatic story.

IN DRAMATIC PLAY, LET YOUR CHILD BE THE DIRECTOR, CREATING CHARACTERS AND DETERMINING PLOT. THEN WATCH FOR WHAT ROLE YOU SHOULD PLAY.

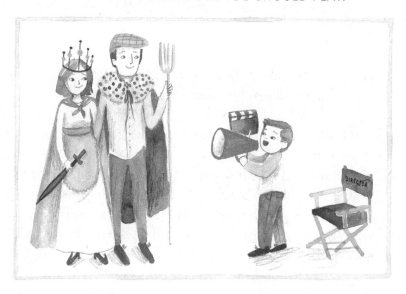

In this case, you're watching specifically for emotional cues regarding what's going on in the pretend-play scenario. Consider which feelings might be motivating the characters' action. Name feelings when you can, guided by the context and by what your child does, but stay focused simply on observing and attuning. This is the expressive play approach we discussed above.

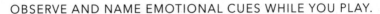

OBSERVE AND NAME EMOTIONAL CUES WHILE YOU PLAY.

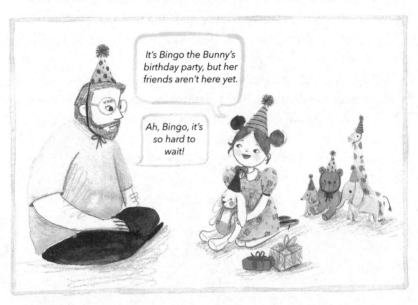

Again, you're not taking the lead. You're just watching and listening, then giving emotional cues about what you observe.

Step 2: If invited, act out your part by adding some emotion to your character
Once the dramatic play begins, your child may give you some direction. If so, jump in and, as the character you're playing, make a point of explicitly pointing to the emotions in the story. If you're not sure, just make a guess, drawing from what you'd think a person might feel in that particular situation.

ACT OUT YOUR PART BY ADDING SOME EMOTION TO YOUR CHARACTER.

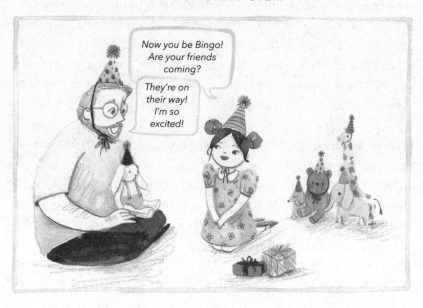

ACT OUT YOUR PART BY ADDING SOME EMOTION TO YOUR CHARACTER.

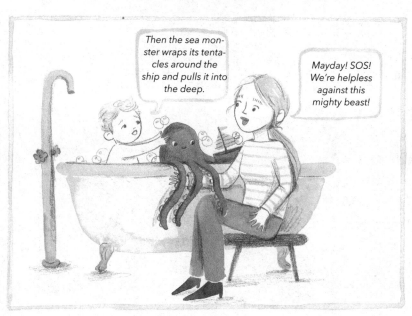

Notice that it's not required that you explicitly name an emotion each time you act out your part. Often you will, and with young children doing so can be especially effective in terms of helping them learn to name their distinctive emotions. But at times it's just fine to act out the emotion—the child will know what you're getting at. The main thing is that you are including and emphasizing the emotions inherent in the scene, both verbally and nonverbally.

Step 3: If you're not offered a character to play, touch on emotions as the narrator

Sometimes your child won't assign you a character to play, or they'll take a character back. In that case, you can just play the role of the narrator of the scene. When that happens, you still want to emphasize the feelings and emotions of the characters in the situation being acted out.

One warning about joining in your child's dramatic play: Avoid being too scary or sad as you act out different scenarios. Yes, you want your child to experience emotions, but the overall goal is to let them do so in the context of a happy, fun, safe interaction with you.

BRING EMOTIONS TO LIFE AS A NARRATOR.

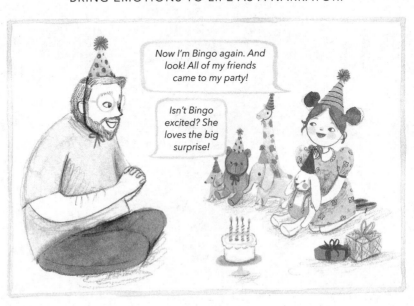

BRING EMOTIONS TO LIFE AS A NARRATOR.

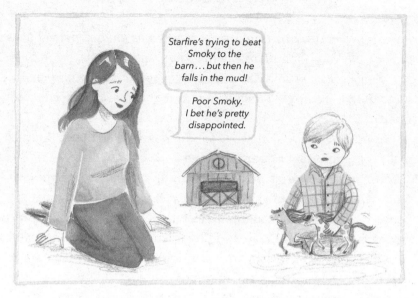

The limbic region, along with the whole nervous system, will read even pretend fear or nervousness or sadness similar to the real thing, so find ways to approach those feelings without allowing your kids to move into disturbing or upsetting emotional places.

BRING EMOTIONS TO LIFE AS A NARRATOR.

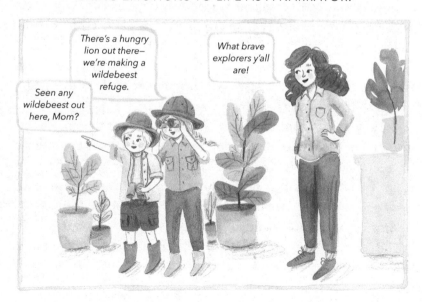

Oh Yes, I'm the Great Pretender

Right now you may be thinking, *I see why this kind of pretend play can be really good for my kids, but that's not at all my thing. I'm just not into giving voice to stuffed animals, or singing like a pop sensation, or pretending to be an NFL player. And acting like I actually enjoy it? Good luck.*

We get it. As we've said, we've felt the same way at times. But this really is as important as we're claiming it is.

Most parents understand that very young kids go through the pretend stage, also known as *symbolic play*. It usually starts sometime between a child's second and third birthdays, when they begin using an object to represent a real-world experience, such as feeding a doll with a cup, and ends when your growing kid decides it's no longer cool to play house. That's an enormous chunk of childhood—up to ten years—devoted to pretending.

There's a reason pretending is such a *thing*. For decades, research has demonstrated that pretend play supercharges developmental domains that promote important abilities in kids: social skills (*I'm the shopkeeper, how can I help you?*), self-esteem (*I'm good at building castles—maybe one day I'll be an architect*), cognitive skills (*Where's my magic wand? Oh, I remember, I left it at Grandma's. I'll get it next weekend*), motor skills (*Who spilled the fairy glitter? Let's pick it up*), and language (*What's another word for a bank robber? A thief!*). Experts agree that pretend play satisfies children's developmental thirst for knowledge at a stage when experience-driven learning is what a child's emotional brain needs most.

Yet as you know, it can often be hard for a parent to join the dramatic play. The truth is, our adult brains evolved past the pretend stage, and now we have highly developed executive structures in the upper cortical areas that help us attend to the serious business of work and parenting, helping us direct and guide our kids mostly by lending our older, wiser cortex, as we covered previously. A parent's brain is exquisitely attuned to so many details that it's easiest for us to take a more top-down approach to just about everything, using language and logic in ways that make sense to us but that just aren't how our children most intuitively go about things.

So when it comes time for dramatic play, the best thing you can do is to combine your logic-based thinking with your emotional wisdom. You know, on a rational level, that pretend play offers countless benefits for your kids. And your emotional wisdom leads you to want what's best for them. Just like your child gets better at the things they practice, you'll get better at playing, and it will get easier. So even though it might not always feel completely natural, jump in! You don't have to be perfect, or even especially good at it. Don't overthink it. Have some fun! Your kids will love having you play with them and follow their lead into pretend worlds unknown.

> Even though it might not always feel completely natural, jump in! You don't have to be perfect, or even especially good at it. Don't overthink it. Have some fun! Your kids will love having you play with them and follow their lead into pretend worlds unknown.

There's no doubt about it: Our kids will experience anger, fear, despair, hurt, frustration, regret, and shame. Meltdowns happen. It takes time, and repetition, for children to develop the brain circuitry for calmer thinking and self-control. But negative emotions are temporary states of being—little storms, if you will. It's the parent who knows how to hold and accept the storm, trusting that the feelings will pass, who can guide their child toward peaceful resolution. And as you position yourself to accept the way your child feels with grace and confidence, you may also uncover deeper experiences that are sometimes hidden behind kids' surface behaviors and attitudes, often much more vulnerable feelings that can be teased out with gentleness and subtlety.

If your child is showing undesirable behavior, something more tender usually lies beneath. Once these softer emotions can be accessed and brought to life, you may then share new awareness, insight, and skills that will be easier for kids to adopt, because they'll be so engaged and energized by this stronger and more satisfying emotional bond. That's when they'll be willing and able to make better decisions, even when they're upset.

The research is crystal clear: We can have an enormous influence on the way our children learn to deal with emotions. When we allow feelings to emerge, or come to life, as emotions that can be recognized as part of who our children are—and who they are becoming—we begin to view those emotions not as problems but rather as powerful tools for positive change, mature growth, and relational connection.

So use playtime with your kids to help them learn to bring their emotions to life, which means recognizing their feelings, expressing what's going on inside themselves, dealing with fears and anxieties that have cropped up, and acting in ways that lead to better overall behavior. When these skills get combined with the self-awareness and empathy produced by the earlier PlayStrong strategies, your children will be well on their way to living lives full of meaning, significance, and relational connection.

> We can have an enormous influence on the way our children learn to deal with emotions.

Dial Intensity Up or Down

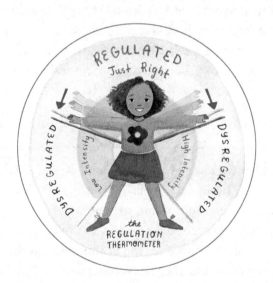

Primary skill being developed in the child:
An ability to regulate their emotions and actions when
they're upset and struggling.

Primary message received by the child:
Someone is going to be here for me when I'm out of control
and can't handle things very well by myself.

By now you're beginning to build quite the play-based parental tool kit. We've introduced you to the Think Out Loud strategy and how you can use play to teach your kids about their internal worlds so they can gain a fuller sense of what's going on in their minds. With Make Yourself a Mirror, you've learned ways you can help them build a fuller and deeper understanding of their emotional lives and how to use that knowledge to interact and connect with others on a more meaningful level. And in Bring Emotions to Life, you've seen how those earlier lessons can lead kids to better regulate their emotions and behaviors, express what's going on inside them, and make better decisions. As you play with your kids and help them develop these various skills, you're also sending clear and important messages that someone sees and understands them at a deep level, and that they have the ability to notice, manage, and express their emotions.

Now let's turn to our next PlayStrong strategy, Dial Intensity Up or Down, which focuses on how play can help our children when they're having a hard time, and what we as caregivers can do when we see them getting out of control or having big emotional responses.

Chase the Why

Take a second and imagine your kid, or one of your kids. See them in your mind's eye. Envision them playing, having fun. Now think about times when that play stops going so well. Maybe they get too rambunctious or even aggressive and seem too intense and out of control. Or maybe it's the opposite, and at times they seem checked out or shut down, almost like they're avoiding joining in an activity with other kids or failing to match what's going on around them. Possibly they're upset or they feel overwhelmed in some way.

When our kids are upset, one of the first steps we should aim to take is to respond with curiosity. As Tina has said for decades, "Chase the why." *Why are they throwing a tantrum (or whining, or quitting the game, or yelling at a sibling) right now?* When children act in some way that we don't like, parents are often tempted to immediately move to punishment of some kind. And while we're big proponents of setting clear boundaries for kids, we strongly believe that before responding in any way, parents should start by being curious about *why* their kid is acting this way. You might eventually decide that discipline is in order.

A quick aside: Discipline should always be about teaching, not punishment. Yes, set boundaries and enforce limits. Kids need that. But the point of discipline is *not* to punish or give consequences. It's to help children learn where the parameters lie and build skills to make better decisions next time, or over time, as development unfolds. Make this priority the point of your discipline. And before you discipline, or address the behavior in any way, get curious—chase the why—about what might be going on with your child in this moment.

Remember, behavior is communication, so by watching how your children respond to various play-based situations, you can better understand what their actions are telling you, and then you can be responsive and help them when they become upset and behave in ways that aren't optimal. It might look like your son is having a furious reaction to his big brother because he doesn't want to share a Lego tower he built, but if you chase the why beyond surface behaviors, you might discover that he doesn't want his brother to break it because he's giving the tower to Grandma and he wants it to be really tall for her, and he needs your help to protect something he created.

Or you might think that your daughter wants to quit the soccer team she begged to sign up for because she just won't work hard, but it might be that she's overwhelmed walking up to a group of kids at practice and games. So she might need you to get her there a bit earlier so she can slowly warm up and receive kids as they arrive instead of having to enter an already-gathered group. When you first chase the why, you can more quickly address the challenging situation in the moment—by dialing intensity up or down—and help your child build skills that prevent the situation from happening as often in the future.

When you first chase the why, you can more quickly address the challenging situation in the moment—by dialing intensity up or down—and help your child build skills that prevent the situation from happening as often in the future.

And it's not only behavior that communicates. Your child's various sensitivities and preferences are full of important information about what's going on with them as well. To a significant degree, kids' play preferences are rooted in their sensory systems. They seek out information by moving, seeing, feeling, smelling, tasting, and touching, and the types of play they do or don't enjoy can tell us much about how they're wired and why they're behaving as they are. Your child might love running or jumping, or they might feel most comfortable hanging upside down from the jungle gym. Or perhaps they love to be smushed between two giant pillows. Some kids get excited by spinning around, and others can't stand being dizzy. Some enjoy big, loud, echoing spaces, while for others, these feel almost scary. Some love big sights, sounds, and smells, whereas others become easily overwhelmed by them. Kids seek more of whatever they love to do or feel.

And likewise, whatever makes them feel icky or uncomfortable, they tend to avoid. A child's play tells us a lot about their strengths and sensitivities as they interact with others and their environment. Sometimes they desire more intensity; sometimes less. You likely already have a good sense of some of your child's sensory preferences, starting from when they were a tiny infant. Some babies calm quickly with slow bouncing and swaying, and other babies love being moved and swayed with more gusto. Your baby may have been calmed from a snug swaddle, whereas others, like Tina's best friend, got nicknamed Baby Born-free because she didn't like anything constrictive in her infant and toddler years.

Our fourth PlayStrong strategy, Dial Intensity Up or Down, is all about focusing in on your child's behavior and sensory preferences and using what you observe to help them make better decisions regarding their choices and actions—all while building self-regulation skills for the future. Using this strategy can help you create more robust circuitry between your child's body and parts of the brain called the somatosensory cortex and the motor cortex. These neurological components are largely responsible for directing the orchestra of information that allows kids to sit and listen, wait their turn, pay attention, hand objects over gently, use the right amount of force, and play safely and carefully. This strategy is about attuning to your kids during their play so you can notice their level of emotional and physical intensity in a situation and, if necessary, dial it up or down depending on what's called for in that moment.

> This strategy is about attuning to your kids during their play so you can notice their level of emotional and physical intensity in a situation and, if necessary, dial it up or down depending on what's called for in that moment.

Your Child's Regulation Thermostat

Picture a traditional thermostat, the kind we used before everything went digital.

THE REGULATION THERMOSTAT.

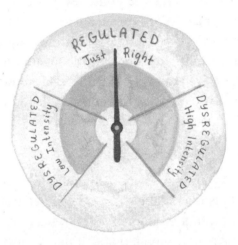

Look at the region at the top of the thermostat labeled "regulated." That's where kids are when things are going well. They're able to make good decisions and handle themselves appropriately. They might feel silly or excited, or they might even be sad or disappointed, but when they're in a regulated state, they can still maintain control of their emotions and actions. Even if they experience anxiety, frustration, anger, or some other strong negative emotion, they'll be able to remain regulated and, for the most part, remain in charge of the way they behave.

But obviously, no child is able to remain regulated all the time. Sensory challenges arise and may cause an intense and often emotional reaction. It might be because high energy or increased sensory input has pervaded the environment, in the form of noise or something else. That can rev some kids up and create an especially intense reaction to a situation, where they become too dialed up and end up losing control as their nervous systems try to modulate the energy in the room.

Or, for other kids, it can move them in the other direction on the dial, causing them to tend toward being too dialed down. They might withdraw literally and physically, or they might go silent and implicitly remove themselves from the interactions with the others in the situation. They might lock themselves in their room or just shut down and refuse to respond when someone tries to help or converse with them. In both dysregulated states, whether the child's response is too activated or not activated enough, they are dysregulated, reactive, and unable to handle themselves well as they deal with challenging and unpredictable moments.

Finding Sensory Regulation

Let's get more specific about what can create regulation or dysregulation in kids. Numerous factors can rev kids up too much or cause them to shut down, and one of the most powerful dynamics at play has to do with their sensory preferences.

Sensory integration processing is a sophisticated interplay of multiple physical input systems that allow us to act and react appropriately to a particular situation. We all know about the five basic body senses (sight, hearing, taste, smell, touch), but there are other, less obvious senses that you may not be aware of: the vestibular sense (having to do with the inner ear and detecting changes in your balance or body orientation when you go upside down or spin around), proprioception (related to the signals from your muscles and joints about your body position in space), and interoception (associated with the internal signals your body sends, such as when you're hungry, you need to go to the bathroom, or you experience a particular emotional state).

Often occurring beneath conscious, surface-level behavior, sensory processing directs the flow of information among the environment, the brain, and the nervous system in a bottom-up way. How our sensory system processes and integrates information can sometimes be out of sync. It can be under-responsive, over-responsive, or both, creating too much or not enough intensity—or a vacillation back and forth. Either extreme typically results in all kinds of challenges, such as behavioral, attentional, academic, and social issues.

Unique differences in sensory processing can greatly impact a child's social interactions (among other things), making them more and less naturally enjoyable to be around. In other words, sensory awareness and integration can help your child enjoy closer, more satisfying interactions where all play partners feel understood and their boundaries respected, or the lack of it can create social turbulence, reactivity, more frequent misunderstandings, and greater conflict.

> Sensory awareness and integration can help your child enjoy closer, more satisfying interactions where both play partners feel understood and their boundaries respected, or the lack of it can create social turbulence, reactivity, more frequent misunderstandings, and greater conflict.

Every child will become dysregulated, losing their sensory and emotional balance, and they'll do so on a fairly regular basis—especially in their early years. We can't expect otherwise. The key is to help them stay regulated as often as possible, and to co-regulate, or help them return to regulation when their intensity gets dialed too high or too low. Then, over time, we want to give them skills that, as they mature, they can use to regulate *themselves* when they begin to lose control. Children develop the emotional agility to regulate themselves via lots of repeated experiences where we, the adults in their lives, help co-regulate them. We let them "borrow" our regulation, helping calm down their nervous systems with our peaceful, supportive presence. Ultimately, the goal is to expand kids' ability to remain comfortable there at the top of the intensity thermostat. That's what this PlayStrong strategy is all about.

> **P**arental Goals for Children's Sensory and Emotional Intensity:
>
> · Help kids *remain* regulated.
> · Help kids *return* to regulation when they've left it.
> · Help kids *expand* their ability to remain regulated.

Sensory Seekers and Sensory Avoiders

There are different ways to categorize and understand sensory preferences, but for simplicity's sake, we can say that, generally, children fall into one of two categories. Some are *sensory seekers*. They have a high threshold, and even a *need,* for sensory input and physical sensations, whether in the form of touch, noise, smells, speed, spinning, movement, or something else. They might love loud music or wrestling and rolling on the floor. Or they enjoy clomping through the house using noisy, heavy steps, and they might even experience an unusual tolerance for pain.

Others, in contrast, are *sensory avoiders*. Their threshold for sensory input is low. They feel uncomfortable in loud spaces and often get overwhelmed at parties and on playdates. Hugs and kisses may not really be their thing, and they'll often have difficulty wearing clothes that feel scratchy or tight to them.

Most parents, not knowing about sensory input, see sensory avoidance—like refusing to get dressed or having major meltdowns when it's time to bathe and get their hair wet—as oppositional or disobedient. However, when we chase the why, a more informed look tells us that their systems simply can't always manage the input they receive, leaving them easily overwhelmed. They're uncomfortable, and their behaviors are attempts to feel more comfortable. Understandable. They're trying to make their world work for them. Keep in mind that certain types of sensory input—smells, sounds, textures, tastes—can be perceived as a cue of *threat* in their nervous systems, so we may even see fight, flight, and freeze types of responses.

> Would you describe your child as more sensory seeking or sensory avoiding? Understanding the difference can go a long way toward knowing why they get overwhelmed and how best to help them when they become upset.

One important caveat: It's not the case that children fit into one category at the exclusion of the other. For example, a child might be more sensory seeking when it comes to one particular preference (they might enjoy pushing and crashing into people and things) but then also sensory avoidant for another sense (they don't like to touch gooey stuff or might be a picky eater).

So it's not the case that one child can be exclusively characterized as *either* sensory seeking or sensory avoiding. Instead, those tendencies are just what the word says: tendencies. In one context and moment, the child might be more sensitive to sensory inputs. But when circumstances change, so might the child's unique sensory preferences. And when stressors—moving, family visiting, loss of a pet, divorce—are added to the mix, it can shift or intensify sensory preferences even more. On the flip side, when de-stressors—play, feeling safe, feeling connected, being in nature, having enough sleep—are made readily available, we can see shifts *away from* sensory sensitivity to more sensory tolerance and resilience.

We all have sensory preferences, and at times they don't match up with what our partner or child prefers. Tina, for example, loves to have all the curtains open and the lights on. Her sons, on the other hand, must have inherited vampire genes somewhere down the line—they actually *prefer* that their rooms stay dimly lit. (Their vampire ancestors apparently didn't have a sensory aversion to significant messiness, either!)

Sometimes that's just the case: The sensory profiles of parent and child don't match up very well. If a child is sensory seeking and wants to be in Mom's lap all the time, and if Mom is typically more sensory averse and gets "touched out" easily, a collision of sensory needs can occur. When there are co-parents, it's usually the case that one parent can better relate than the other to the sensory profile of a child. The key is to notice and be aware of our own and our child's sensory preferences so that we can intentionally make efforts to get those needs met instead of constantly reacting against each other.

One note regarding the moments we're not at our best as parents: Family life can be loud, chaotic, smelly, and really overwhelming. When we reflect on some of the times we were less patient as parents, we come to see that our impatience and reactivity may have been primarily from sensory overload and feeling overwhelmed. What a great thing to learn about ourselves, and to notice our sensory gauges so we can tend to our own nervous systems and give ourselves what we might need, like some quiet, to feel more regulated.

As you become more aware of your child's sensory system's preferences, sensitivities, and needs (and your own), you can provide more input or stimuli from a different, complementary sensory mode that will have a more regulating effect on your child. Use one sense to turn up or down another.

Imagine, for example, that your toddler is stirring dirt and water to make mud pies, and she loves the tactile feeling of water on her skin so much that she begins vigorously splashing brown water everywhere, including on you. Or she's just so enthused about seeking sensations that it's making her motor control all wonky. Stuff is flying everywhere because her dial is so turned up on the tactile sense that she's not able to be totally in charge of her body right now. In this instance, let's also imagine that your preferred sensory mode is the opposite. She's in heaven splattered in mud, but you feel mildly ill just looking at the brown goop.

Instead of just telling her to stop, turn up a different sensory mode to counteract the mode that's run amok or is conflicting with yours. You could offer to add a big bucketful of dirt to make the mud pies thicker and heavier, then hand her a giant heavy spoon to stir it with. You've just introduced a new stream of more proprioceptive (or "push-pull") input that will encourage her to slow down and work harder with the thicker substance. Sure, she'll probably want to squish her hands in it, too, because she's a tactile seeker at heart, but at least there will be a smaller amount of yucky water splashing all over!

The point is that it's important to have a good sense of who your kid is and to be able to notice and name—to Think Out Loud—their overall mental and emotional state when you're interacting with or observing them. The more and better you can pay attention to their sensory preferences, the more adept you'll be at recognizing when things seem out of whack—or even better, are *about* to go in that direction—and then engaging with your child in the way they need you to, whether that's by turning the dial up or turning it down.

> The more and better you can pay attention to their sensory preferences, the more adept you'll be at recognizing when things seem out of whack—or even better, are *about* to go in that direction—and then engaging with your child in the way they need you to, whether that's by turning the dial up or turning it down.

Parents as Co-regulators

There are ways you can join in play with your kids that develop their ability to self-regulate by paying attention to what's happening in their bodies and what they need to do to adjust and achieve a state of balance. But this is a skill that you need to help them build. In other words, children aren't born knowing how to regulate themselves. We are their first co-regulators.

> Children aren't born knowing how to regulate themselves. We are their first co-regulators.

For some physical sensations, this comes pretty naturally for most parents. When our children are babies, we might adjust a blanket or cool down a room if their body temperature is running too cold or hot; that's an example of acting as an early sensory regulator. Then, as they get older, kids learn how to detect those changes and become better *self*-regulators, knowing to put on or take off a sweatshirt, for example. Along the way, they get better at recognizing more subtle nuances beyond more obvious sensations like body temperature. They learn to expect where their energy level should be and how they should control their bodies when, for example, they're reading in the library, or playing tag with friends, or jumping in a party bounce house full of other kids. Self-regulation involves monitoring what's happening in their bodies and directing mental attention where it needs to flow so that they can know what's going on, switch on greater awareness, detect subtle changes, and act intentionally to make adjustments to calm or regain focus and a sense of control. They can dial things up or down as necessary.

Children look to parent responses to sensory input as cues of safety and threat, as well. If, when you get sand on your hands, you immediately wipe them off, grimace, and say how much you hate being dirty, your child will pay attention to that response. If, when the doorbell rings, you startle, gasp, and look worried, your child might think that it's an unsafe noise rather than one that indicates a fun package or social engagement. This isn't to say that you can always temper your sensory responses, especially if you tend to be more of a sensory seeker or sensory avoider yourself. But your awareness of your responses and how your child might be reading your cues can significantly affect how they interact with their own environment and the people around them.

As with the other PlayStrong strategies, this process takes time, and we have to be patient as development unfolds and as kids learn from lots of experiences. In the meantime, we need to act as the external co-regulators. Again, the way children learn to self-regulate is by having many, many experiences of their parent providing the kind of connection and co-regulation that lets their nervous system practice what it's like to recognize dysregulation, then move from there back to regulation. As their brain gets lots of reps, or repeated experiences, of having their parents help them become more regulated by dialing intensity up or down, their brains wire for how to move from a dysregulated state to a regulated state, and they do so for themselves. Self-regulation is built from co-regulation experiences.

Dial Intensity Up or Down: Step by Step

What, specifically, does that mean, to be a child's co-regulator?

Regulation is about the ability to get back into a state of balance. When we're talking about co-regulation, we mean that we are providing our presence to join with our child to guide them and support them as they return to a state of regulation. Dan Siegel describes regulation as "monitoring and modifying." So, that means watching for opportunities to tune in to our child's state and help them modify it—dialing up or down your child's emotional state when necessary. Right now we're focusing on play specifically, but as with all of the other PlayStrong strategies, this one applies to other, non-play moments when your child becomes dysregulated. (More on this to come.)

There are specific steps you can take to encourage emotional and sensory balance and help your child return to a "just right" spot on their intensity thermostat. Instead of immediately shutting down emotionally intense behavior or pushing and prodding kids when their energy and engagement are too low, you can take practical steps to help them match their sensory state to the demands of the situation, thus easing them back toward regulation.

> Instead of immediately shutting down emotionally intense behavior or pushing and prodding kids when energy and engagement are too low, you can take practical steps to help them match their sensory state to the demands of the situation, thus easing them back toward regulation.

And that's the key—*easing* them back. Notch by notch: That's your goal. You'll rarely be able to quickly move a kid from dysregulation to regulation. But every notch in that direction makes things more pleasant for each of you and makes it that much easier for them to move back toward the "just right" section of the dial.

The practical steps for PlayStrong strategy #4 are similar to the steps you've been learning in the other strategies. Once again, the strategy begins with paying attention and attuning to your child and what's going on in their mind.

Step 1: Observe and attune, watching for signs that they might be becoming dysregulated

It's really not too difficult to see when a child is becoming dysregulated on the "too intense" side of the scale, especially if you've been watching for what their sensory preferences are. The signs are fairly obvious. Is the child . . .

- Moving too fast?
- Being too loud?

- Playing too rough?
- Being excessively silly?
- Putting non-food items in their mouth?
- Touching everything in sight?
- Appearing overstimulated?
- Having difficulty transitioning activities?
- Feeling or expressing anger or big emotions in ways that feel out of sync with the situation or the people around them?

When you see evidence of any of the above, there's a decent chance that your child is becoming too revved up (or that they've already passed their point).

Low-intensity attributes aren't nearly as raucous and boisterous, but they're fairly easy to spot as well. During playtime, is your child . . .

- Moving too slowly?
- Being too quiet or withdrawn?
- Pouting, refusing to continue playing?
- Seeming bored, uninterested, or lethargic?
- Feeling or expressing sadness that doesn't seem to match the circumstances?
- Appearing understimulated?
- Shutting down and avoiding sensory input?
- Removing themself from a game after becoming upset?

If so, then most likely their intensity level has moved to a level that's too low.

For this first step, all you're doing is observing and attuning, watching your child's behaviors and looking for any information that can help you respond to what the child needs.

Step 2: Chase the why

Once you get a sense of how they're acting and what it might be telling you about their level of dysregulation, it's time to get curious. What's going on with them right now? What set them off? What is their sensory need right now?

Do they feel embarrassed that they didn't perform better in the game? Are they angry that their sister blurted out the joke's punch line before they could tell it? Are they unwilling to share? Do they feel overwhelmed by all the commotion?

Sometimes they're frustrated that they can't be more proficient in an activity they love, and they react with anger, possibly even taking their emotions out on you.

BEFORE RESPONDING WHEN KIDS GET UPSET, CHASE THE WHY.

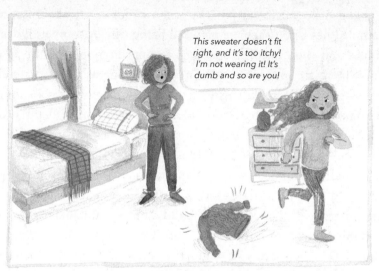

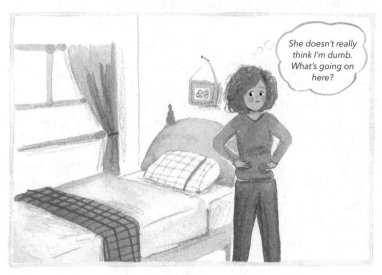

Curiosity can be a revelatory approach to take when your kid is upset. If you'll simply chase the why, you'll be amazed at how much information you'll discover and how useful that data can be as you try to move your child back into a regulated emotional state.

Step 3: Dial the intensity up or down

Remember, the goal is to help kids avoid one extreme or the other, and instead to stay in the center of the thermostat while they play—and to practice how to find regulation in other situations as well.

This can be particularly tricky when children play because, for example, they often vacillate between being silly or competitive one minute and then needing space or feeling disappointed the next. When there are more intense sensory components to play, such as lots of spinning, or playing with something slimy, or screaming, maintaining a state of regulation often becomes more difficult. Over time, we want to help expand their ability to remain in control of their emotions in order to meet the demands of the situation.

After all, when kids are in an emotional and sensory state where they can remain regulated as they play, they'll be better able to engage with others, learn new skills, and build more coordinated patterns of movement and communication. They'll also be able to access progressively higher levels of regulating and relating and therefore expand the extent to which they can handle themselves well when things don't go their way. They can manage and respond to their emotions and prevent their regulation from going off the rails toward a chaotic, overwhelmed stress reaction of overstimulation, or a rigid, checked-out, understimulated state.

Let's be clear, though: We're not saying that you help your kid avoid any negative emotion whatsoever, or that you should perfectly curate a tailored sensory environment every moment. For example, you might notice that they're looking sad because they've been left out of an experience; maybe they're sitting with their head down, possibly even with a tear or two, arms crossed and not wanting to talk.

In a situation like this, we're not suggesting that you should start cheerleading and trying to get them happy in that moment. Giving your children opportunities to feel their feelings when the emotions are healthy and appropriate is one of the best things you can do to help them learn the skills of emotional resilience. (More on this in the next chapter.)

Remember, the brain gets better at what we practice. So when kids feel overwhelmed by the sensory environment, or sad, or angry, or anxious, and you show up in the moment to listen and comfort and be present to their experience, you're giving them practice at dealing with unpleasant emotions, with you there at their side. And then, when it's time to move out of that moment to begin to play again or shift into another state, that's a brain-building moment as well, and we want to optimize it by helping them move back toward regulation.

The process is fairly simple (if not always easy to do):

When kids are running too hot or too cold, our job is (1) to co-regulate with our calm presence and support, and then (2) to provide sensory inputs that help move them back toward regulation. And the inputs you offer might be about calming things down or revving things up.

Let's talk about this process more specifically.

Cooling Things Off: Dialing Intensity Down

While some intensity is regulating for some children, when a child gets upset or becomes *too* intense or aggressive while they're playing, we typically need to help them dial the intensity down. But if you're like most parents, you may find that sometimes you end up counter-productively dialing it up instead.

In the illustrations that follow, see how these parents dialed down the intensity in their second examples? Notice that, instead of using a top-down strategy like lecturing the child or trying to convince them to immediately act differently, both parents started from the bottom up. They helped their kids calm down through co-regulation by comforting them, connecting with them, and using a soothing tone of voice to lower the intensity of the situation. (The mom with

INSTEAD OF DIALING THE INTENSITY EVEN HIGHER . . .

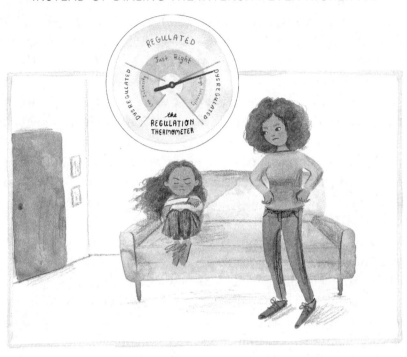

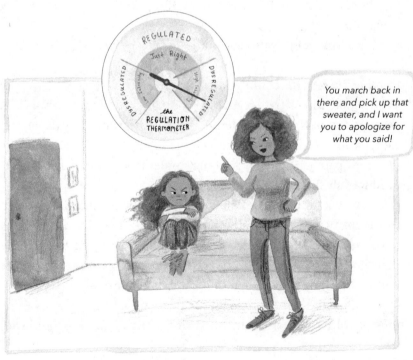

DIAL THE INTENSITY DOWN AND HELP YOUR CHILD
REGAIN REGULATION.

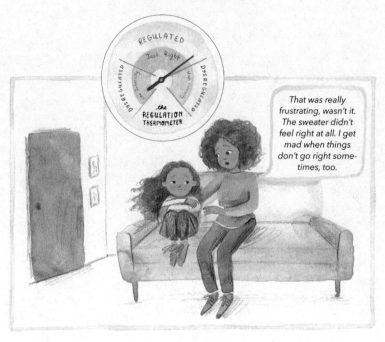

THEN, WHEN YOUR CHILD HAS CALMED, HANDLE ANY DISCIPLINE
(WHICH IS ALL ABOUT TEACHING AND BUILDING SKILLS).

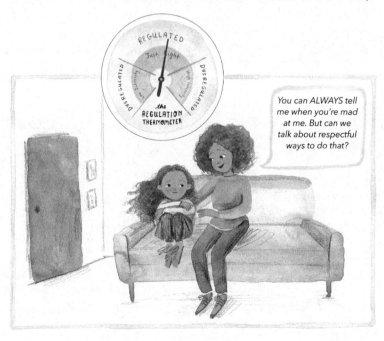

INSTEAD OF DIALING THE INTENSITY EVEN HIGHER . . .

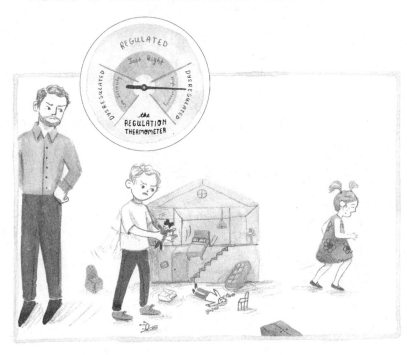

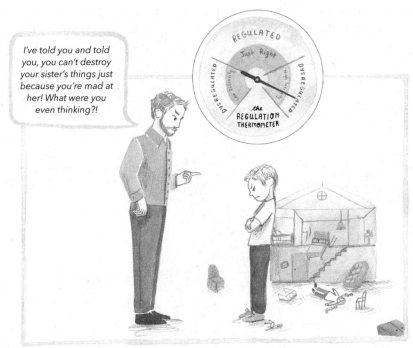

DIAL THE INTENSITY DOWN AND HELP YOUR CHILD REGAIN REGULATION.

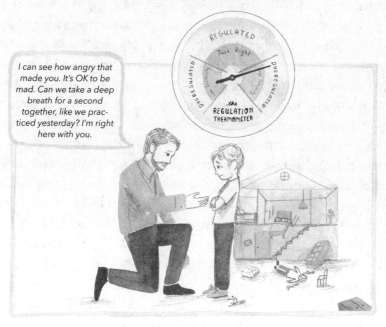

THEN, WHEN YOUR CHILD HAS CALMED, HANDLE ANY DISCIPLINE (WHICH IS ALL ABOUT TEACHING AND BUILDING SKILLS).

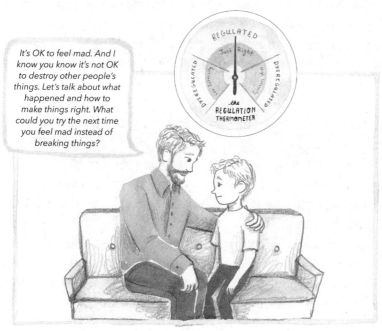

the "dumb" sweater found her daughter huddled on the sofa and helped calm her with gentle touch.) Then, once the kids were regulated enough to hear and process new information, the parents could be more effective in the discipline (teaching) process and use language and problem-solving, which is more top down, to help their kids understand and think about the lessons they wanted to teach. (We'll talk a lot more about limit setting and discipline in an upcoming strategy, in case you want more help with that process.)

There's an almost infinite number of bottom-up strategies you can use to help a child become more regulated when things begin to get out of hand. For example, imagine that you and your young son are pirates at the moment, fencing with foam swords on the deck of your ship. But soon, he begins to hit you harder and harder. He doesn't mean anything by it, and he's not angry, but his sensory-seeking desires have resulted in a high level of aggression, and he's lost any awareness of your experience. What he needs in this moment is to have you help him dial back his intensity so he can down-regulate and move back into a calmer state.

We're not saying that it's inherently wrong to say something like, "Not so hard!" And again, boundaries are important for kids. In fact, it's important that we do so. But there are so many better options than reacting with an instinctive "Stop it!" or "No!" After all, in many situations, as in this case, you simply need to adjust the intensity, not completely stop the action immediately. So if you can just dial things down a bit, the game can continue and you two can get back to enjoying each other. "Medium" is a wonderfully descriptive way to ease down the dial and realistically ask the child to modulate his use of force. It's almost an impossible expectation for him to go from hard to gentle. But if you pause and show him how medium feels by pressing the sword against his arm, he can more likely adjust to that level of intensity.

By combining this bottom-up approach, where you let him feel the different pressure in his body, with the top-down explanation about using medium force, you'll be much more likely to be effective in getting your son to tone down his bodily actions in response to his sensory needs.

DIAL DOWN THE INTENSITY BY DECREASING THE FORCE.

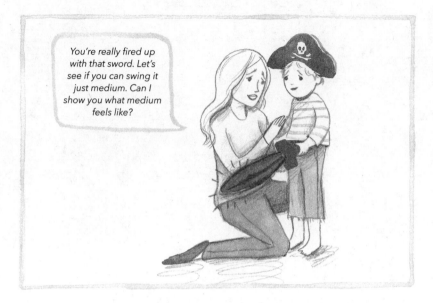

That's only one example of how you can dial down the intensity in a situation where a child is becoming too intense. Another would be to allow your son to expend energy but lower the effects of his actions. That might mean swapping out the harder foam sword with a softer pool noodle if your son continues to need more proprioceptive sensory input or intense emotional release. Then he can continue to use the same amount of energy and even tire himself out, but he's less likely to hurt you in the process. Or, you can grab a soft pillow as a shield to block and protect your body, replacing aggressive, pain-producing behavior while still letting your son swing the sword with acceptable levels of intensity. Along the way, you might model taking jabs as if with more force but slow down right before contact, so your son can see this alternative during a pretend fight. However you do it, the point is that you're taking the physical intensity and lowering its actual effects. You might even consider taking a break in the play scenario by calling a pirate refueling session—"Let's scavenge the land to see what tasty morsels we can find!"—to get a snack or a drink of water. Then you can start back up when you observe that your child's dial has moved back to the regulation zone.

DIAL DOWN THE INTENSITY BY LOWERING
THE PHYSICAL EFFECTS.

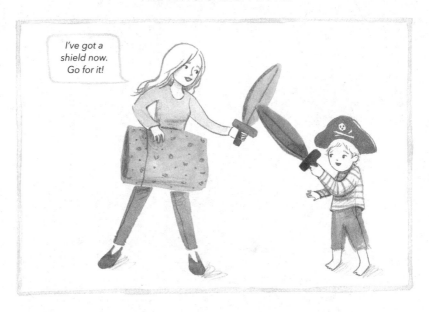

As we discussed in the previous chapter, one of the most powerful tools we always have at our disposal is storytelling, and it can serve as an effective strategy for dialing down intensity. For instance, if your child keeps hitting too hard, driving you back toward a wall as you block the hits with your sword or a pillow shield, you can pull in a storyline, in this case from the pirate narrative you two have going: "Ahoy, matey. I'm getting perilously close to the side of the ship. If I get driven back any farther, I'll be knocked overboard!" Dial down your own intensity in the play at this moment by using a calmer voice with a slower cadence. Doing so will help model what degree of regulation you're expecting from your child. If you dial up your own intensity by fighting back harder or yelling, your child is likely to mirror those emotions.

This scenario forces the child to make a choice: Do I keep hitting this hard and knock my opponent overboard? Or should I back off because I want to keep the action going? Either option offers the potential for dialing down the intensity. If he retreats and gives you a chance to regain your footing on the ship, great. If, on the other hand, he says you're going over the side and keeps coming at you with the sword, then you can fall to the floor, make an "Ahhhhh!" sound on your descent, then pretend to tread water until your son decides to throw you a rope, or let you get carried away by a sea monster, or say you'll end up in the depths of Davy Jones's locker.

Notice that wherever he takes the story, he's now having to engage his logic and make a choice. He must become immediately aware of what his body is doing and make an intentional decision about the plot of the narrative, and that process inevitably leads him back toward using his mind and becoming more regulated.

That said, there may be times when your pirate opponent becomes so taken by dysregulation that this logic component doesn't engage and pushes the play toward something unsafe or destructive. If your attempts to use play to guide the scenario back toward a more regulated state are unsuccessful, then you may need to consider a break in the action to cool things off.

DIAL DOWN THE INTENSITY BY
INJECTING STORYTELLING INTO THE PLAY.

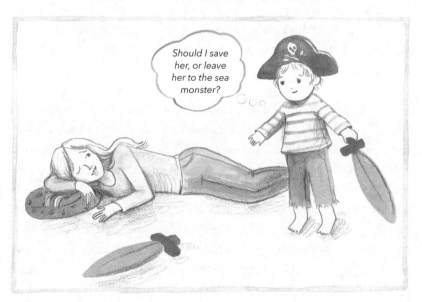

One reminder, for this strategy and for virtually every time you play with your children: Follow their lead. Avoid the temptation to take control of the situation. Instead, give them the upper hand and allow them to take charge. Unless you worry about safety or feel like there's a significant concern that needs to be addressed, let a story play out the way a child wants it to. You might prefer at times that your child show compassion—in this case by tossing you a life preserver. But remember, this is fantasy, and the chief goal in the moment is to enjoy playing, and sometimes that means letting the bad guy (or the good guy, if your child is the villain in the scenario) deal with the results of the climax of the story. In other words, don't force moral and ethical education into every play situation. Let play be play.

On a related note: When play does involve an imaginary battle between you and your child, keep them feeling a sense of control by giving them the upper hand. Match your child's height by bending your knees to stoop down and use less force. The goal, after all, is to make play enjoyable for as long as the child can stay safely regulated, with occasional dips in and out of dysregulation. So your child should never feel overpowered by you, but more evenly matched, allowing them to dictate who's going to win the sword battle. Usually they'll want to retain their power in the end, but regardless, supporting them to stay regulated in a balanced repartee makes everyone a winner.

Bringing More Heat: Dialing Intensity Up

Sometimes the problem isn't that your child's energy is too high in the moment but too low. As before, this typically occurs when a child gets upset or overwhelmed. Maybe they lost a game, or they might feel frustrated because they haven't been able to get you to play the way they want you to. (*That's not how a doctor does it!*) Sometimes the energy in the moment will just get too high for certain kids, and at times things move too fast, leaving them feeling overwhelmed. And just as their intensity might go too high in response, at other times it might completely drop off the table, leaving them shut down or withdrawn.

COMMON LOW-INTENSITY REACTIONS.

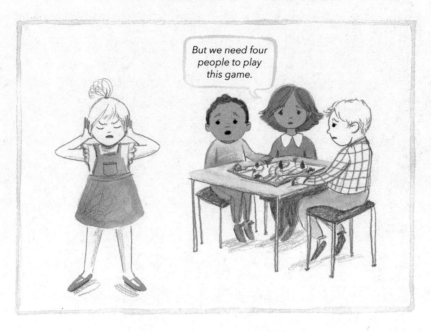

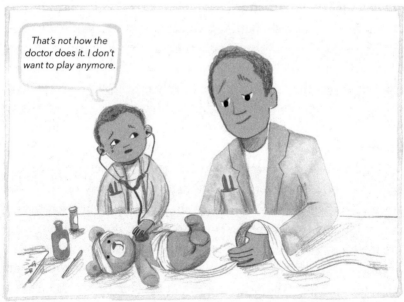

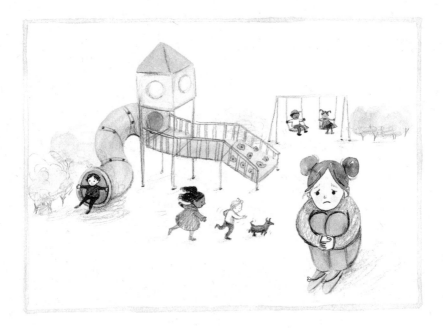

Low-intensity reactions can take many forms, but as a rule, they usually involve the child putting an end to, or at least suspending, the play in one way or another. In contrast to high-intensity situations where the child might explode or become flooded by big, intense emotions, here they would be more likely to withdraw, get quiet, or shut down the play altogether. Some kids even *start* in a low-energy zone because they are slower to warm up or they feel nervousness in a new situation.

Shutting down may occur when they feel overwhelmed and out of control of the circumstances and of themselves. When they feel over-powered or helpless, they will often simply remove themselves from the situation. At times they just need to slow things down and modu-late the state of affairs, so they step away from the action because they simply can't continue to function with that amount of sensory input. We knew one boy who, when he would become dysregulated while playing with his brothers, would climb into the family's dryer and stay there until he calmed down. (No, his brothers never closed the door and started a cycle.) This reaction, where kids shut themselves down, has an infinite number of variations, but what they have in common is that the children become so upset that they momentarily pull away and put an end to the play.

How do you dial the intensity back up, so the child can move back toward emotional regulation? It's all about gently nudging them with options that reengage their senses and allow them to physically and emotionally warm back up to the situation. It's important to remember that when a situation causes your child to feel like shutting down, they can get stuck. So even if they *want* to bounce right back and respond differently, or jump in to solve the problem constructively, they just can't access those faculties right away. And that can be as confusing for them as it might be for us.

> It's important to remember that when a situation causes your child to feel like shutting down, they can get stuck. So even if they *want* to bounce right back and respond differently, or jump in to solve the problem constructively, they just can't access those faculties right away. And that can be as confusing for them as it might be for us.

But here's a key idea that applies especially to low-intensity dysregulation: Kids typically need—and want—your help in dialing the intensity back up so they can return to playing and having fun. At times they may need some space, and some time alone, to calm down and collect themselves. But kids almost always wish they could be more in control of themselves when they've begun to shut down. These states are stress states, and they're uncomfortable and unpleasant for the person experiencing them. They feel overwhelmed or sad, but they don't want to be stuck there for too long. They might tell you to go away, but they eventually want you to follow and help. They demand space, but being alone doesn't feel too good, either. One of the best things you can do is to dial up the intensity just a bit, beginning with small, subtle doses of connection that invite your child's sensory and nervous systems to switch back on so they move back toward regulation. In other words, *start low and go slow*.

Imagine, for example, that in the middle of a family game of Don't Let the Beach Ball Touch the Ground (aka The Floor Is Lava: Beach Ball Edition), your youngest child is the first one to miss, and the ball rolls away. Everyone is hurriedly encouraging her to "Go get it!" in the excitement to keep the game going, but she tearfully wails, "It's not fair!" and goes running out of the room. We need to assume that she's trying to manage her feelings of worry or embarrassment, and because all the sensory overload and mixed-up emotion has gone full tilt, it's sending her spiraling down into those emotions. Therefore, running off represents her best effort to regain control of herself by reducing the sensory information coming her way.

Now's your chance to try the "start low and go slow" method to help your child back into regulation. You might be tempted to go in with logic ("Sweetie, you love that game, and now you're missing out. Does that make any sense?") or with high energy ("Watch out, kiddo! Here comes the monster to get you!"). But while those responses might be perfect in other situations, they're rarely going to be effective with a child who is dysregulated and shut down.

Instead, start low and go slow, becoming a part of the quietness your daughter seeks. Simply let her know you are there to make it more peaceful for her. More safe. You might notice that she's chosen a tiny place to crawl into and hide, perhaps behind a door or under a table. Or maybe she dove under the covers of her bed, where she can disappear into a warm hole. She doesn't realize it in this state of dysregulation, but she's sought out exactly what she needs to climb back out of this emotional state: her very own personal sensory-deprivation tank. That's where you can join her, attuning to her mood and responding to her needs, and then slowly encouraging engagement.

Rather than emphasizing language and logic, you might just offer a sympathetic-sounding "Oh, there you are." Or you might even just sit next to her, possibly putting your hand on her leg, or possibly not, depending on what you know about her sensory preferences. Depending on what she needs, you might even feel like it's better to sit on the floor a couple of feet away, or just outside the door with only part of your body visible to her. Then maybe you say, with an averted gaze, "I'm here when you're ready," or you just take an audible deep breath to signal your presence. With this type of low-and-slow approach, you can reduce her sensory input as she draws on you as her co-regulator—you're there, and available to her, without over-stimulating or intruding on her space. To test if she's ready to re-engage with the game, you might slowly roll the ball toward her to see if she participates.

When your child is deep in a dysregulated state like this, think of your approach as minimizing the sensory field for her, including reducing your own size and volume. She may feel as if she's drowning in sadness, injustice, or helplessness, and she might not even be able to handle the sight of another face or the sound of your voice just yet. Too much input from you, too soon, could flip her right into high-intensity

FOR A CHILD WHO'S SHUT DOWN, LOGIC
MAY NOT BE THE BEST CHOICE.

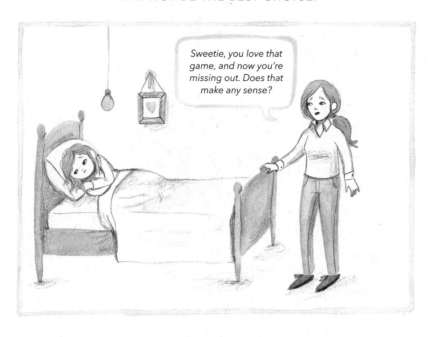

FOR A CHILD WHO'S SHUT DOWN, HIGH ENERGY
MAY NOT BE THE BEST CHOICE.

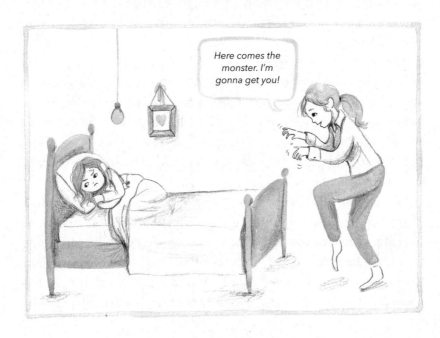

INSTEAD, START LOW AND GO SLOW.

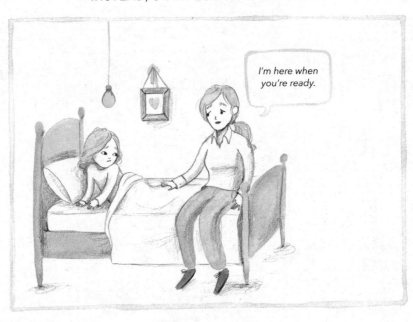

dysregulation, or deeper still into her current state, and that can take longer to work your way out of. So take your time—you might even end up sitting in silence for a couple of awkward minutes—and watch for signs that she could be emerging from her funk, like rustling under the covers, changing her breathing, or peeking to find you.

Along the way, monitor yourself for any free-floating feelings and sensations in your own body. Are you irritated? Anxious to get things moving? Completely unsure of what to do? Whatever you're feeling, you can expect your child to be especially sensitive to it when she's in a low-intensity state. Emotions are contagious, even when she seems shut down or completely checked out, so letting go of feelings you don't need right now can actually help move your child to recover equilibrium more quickly. She's going to come up for air eventually, and when she does, she may need someone to earnestly listen to her account of what happened and how she feels wronged, then to help her weigh other perspectives and offer reassurance that she is indeed wanted in the beach ball game. In so doing, you'll be kindling a small flicker of her awareness and slowly turning up the dial on how much sensory and emotional information she can access, process, and recover from, as you help her return all the way to regulation and back to resuming the game.

Right now you might be asking, *Do I really have to coddle my kid when she's acting out like this? After all, she needs to get used to losing, and it's not fair to her siblings for me to leave the game to nurture her just because she got upset.*

When other kids are involved, that does indeed complicate things a bit. But as long as they're safe and can entertain themselves for a few minutes while you help your daughter, then we promise, even though it might feel counterintuitive, taking a low-and-slow approach with a dysregulated child can not only be the most nurturing thing to do, but it's often more effective. Plus, it's often the quickest way to deal with the situation. The reason is that if you take a couple of minutes to help her regulate, your daughter can then regain equilibrium that much faster. It's not that you're trying to hurry her through her emotions. You're there to help her feel, and then recover.

What's more, especially if you can talk with her later about her reaction, she's going to build skills that will let her better handle similar situations in the future. There's that process again, where co-regulation evolves into self-regulation.

All that said, keep in mind that these strategies aren't magic wands. They're proven to be helpful, and parents have repeatedly told us what a difference they make. Sometimes, though, kids just get upset, and we can't always help them recover right away. They need some time to feel and recuperate. But if you can prioritize these techniques, you'll have a much better chance of helping your children enjoy playing and spend less time in dysregulated states.

And along the way, pay attention to your own regulation dial as well. As we attune to our children and seek to meet them where they are, we may need to adjust our own states to be able to reach them.

A Final Thought: Regulate and Repair

Whether they're exploding or shutting down, whether they're seeking or avoiding sensory stimulation, whether they're toddlers or beginning to look toward tween years and adolescence, whatever age and stage your child is in, play is a powerful tool for helping them learn to regulate their body and nervous system. Then, once they've returned to an equilibrium state of regulation that matches the demands of the situation, it's important that you model for them what it means to reconnect and repair if there are any ruptures within the relationship.

For example, remember the pirate scenario above? Imagine that the mom lost her temper after being hit in the face with the foam sword by her little swashbuckler. (We can all identify with that reaction, can't we?) When it's time to repair, she might use play to make it happen: "Shiver me timbers, Captain, I'm sorry. My emotions were getting the best of me. Can I have a do-over, Captain? Let's make an accord and see what bounty we collected today."

When you model for your kids how to forgive—or, when applicable, how to apologize—then they get to experience that conflict comes and goes, and that things can become good again. Then they can feel safe and know that even when they become upset, they don't have to worry about permanently damaging the relationship. They'll learn to trust, and even expect, that calm and connection will follow conflict. That trust, and that expectation, will serve them extremely well as they grow and develop into teens and adults who face relational challenges even more complex than what to do when both play partners want to wear the Black Panther costume.

So the next time you notice that your child's dial is moving too high or too low, tune in to where they are and to what might be happening to them on a sensory level. Then follow your instincts, along with your knowledge of your child's preferences, to move them back toward a regulated state. You'll be co-regulating, and what's just as important, you'll be taking steps toward helping them self-regulate more and more in the future.

Scaffold and Stretch

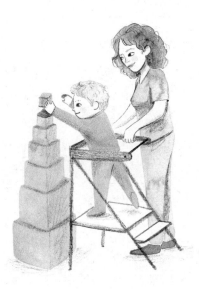

Primary skill being developed in the child:
Resilience in the face of difficult situations.

Primary message received by the child:
Someone is going to show up for me when things get hard,
and I can handle more than I think I can.

Are some kids naturally better than others when it comes to managing stress? Do they just intuitively handle adversity and roll with whatever comes, while others automatically resist new or challenging situations? These questions get at the heart of resilience and grit, two words that mean different things but are fairly interchangeable ways to describe the quality of being able to deal with adversity, bounce back, persist through rough patches, and even learn from obstacles and difficulties. We're talking, in other words, about the ability to handle tough things and keep going.

Based on experiences, development, and personality type, some kids do appear to more naturally embrace challenges with openness, balance, emotional agility, and optimism. It's also the case that resilience and grit are attributes we can build in all of our kids, helping them become more skilled at handling adversity for the rest of their lives. Building these skills is what this PlayStrong strategy, Scaffold and Stretch, is all about. Sometimes kids need supportive scaffolding that will help them deal with difficult issues in the future; and sometimes they need to be stretched to go beyond what's comfortable.

Think for a second about the resilience of your own kids. Are they more likely to avoid challenges whenever possible? Do they seem fragile at times? Do they feel anxious about and resist new experiences, like trying new foods, going away to camp, or singing in a youth choir? Are they ever eager to take up a new hobby or extracurricular activity, only to have their interest fade when they realize it takes more focus and effort than they anticipated?

If you answered yes to any of these questions, that means you've got a kid. Both neurotypical and neurodivergent kids present in these ways at times. Would you like to see them handle themselves differently in certain situations? Sure—at least if you're like virtually every other parent throughout time. But when you see a lack of resilience in your child's actions and reactions, that doesn't mean something's wrong. It just means that development is still in process and that you've found an area where they could use your help building some skills. In this chapter, we want to introduce you to a way of playing that can do just that.

When you see a lack of resilience in your child's actions and reactions, that doesn't mean something's wrong. It just means you've found an area where they could use your help building some skills.

The Value of the Struggle

We'll discuss specific steps for building grit and resilience in just a minute, but first, let's talk about an idea that's absolutely crucial for that process to take place: In order to grow and become emotionally strong, kids need to struggle. They need to be *stretched* beyond what's comfortable. They need to experience a wide range of negative emotions and challenges and discover that they can handle them. When they do, they get practice at regulating their frustrations and anxious feelings well enough to solve problems, both now and in the future. Possibly one of the most amazing skills your child will ever gain is the ability to hold feelings that threaten to topple their composure while maintaining their focus and resolving a difficult issue in front of them.

In order to grow and become emotionally strong, kids need to struggle. They need to be *stretched* beyond what's comfortable. They need to experience a wide range of negative emotions and learn to deal with them. When they do, they get practice at regulating their frustrations and anxious feelings well enough to solve problems, both now and in the future.

Being stretched not only helps children become more proficient in emotional regulation; it also offers them the sweet and rewarding feeling of success once they've overcome challenging obstacles. "I figured it out all by myself" is pure gold in terms of developing a child's internal sense of competence and confidence, which can enliven their desire to take on the next challenge, making it more likely they will take the next steps forward to acquire new skills just beyond their reach. Put this way, then, struggles and even mistakes become iterations toward learning, mastery, and competence.

BUILDING RESILIENCE IS ALL ABOUT EXPANDING A CHILD'S ABILITY TO REGULATE THEMSELF.

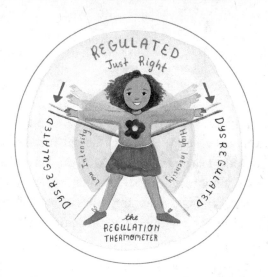

Here's why. When kids choose different tasks where they'll get to try an activity, create something, or take an object apart, more often than not they'll gravitate toward challenges that are within, or pretty close to, their emotional wheelhouse. We can think of that area as their comfort zone. It's the innermost circle in the following diagram, and it represents activities that kids can do by themselves, without help from an adult. The outermost circle we can call the overwhelm zone, and it stands for tasks that ask too much of children. When kids are here, they face challenges they can't meet even with the help of others.

THE ZONE OF PROXIMAL DEVELOPMENT.

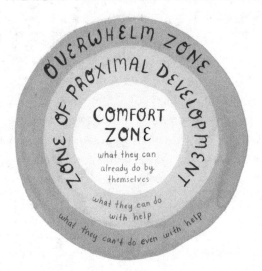

Between these two zones is what developmental experts call the "zone of proximal development" (ZPD).* That's the area where kids are able to competently complete tasks when someone else (like a parent or a teacher) offers specific assistance. The ZPD is where the most learning takes place and where kids can thrive, because here they face what's sometimes called "productive struggle." Here they come up against challenges that stretch them, and since they're not left to handle the obstacles alone, they can achieve success. They have an adult who lets them struggle while also providing the *scaffolding* necessary to accomplish the goal. The ZPD, then, is where we want our kids to spend a good amount of time, since it's here that they're getting both the support and the struggle that can help them grow and learn. They're getting both the scaffolding and the stretching.

As they stretch and try out new abilities during their playtime with you, you'll frequently experience your child bumping up against the edges of the overwhelm zone. That's exactly where you want them to be from time to time, so they can develop more grit and raise their resilience level. Give them enough runway, and enough support, to figure out difficult problems while staying flexible and receptive to

---

* This idea was named and conceptualized by the psychologist Lev Vygotsky.

their emotions—that's how you help expand their ability to remain regulated even in the face of impediments and difficulties.

BY OFFERING YOUR CHILD SCAFFOLDING, THEY CAN STRETCH
BEYOND WHAT THEY THINK THEY CAN ACCOMPLISH.

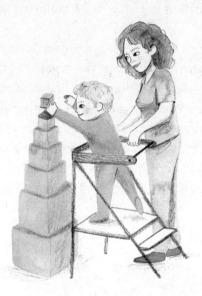

What Keeps Kids from Being More Resilient?

Sometimes, though, rather than helping increase our kids' ability to handle themselves with composure in the face of trouble, we actually do just the opposite. We can point to two main parental tendencies that prevent children from becoming more resilient. First, we don't give them enough opportunities for open-ended play, where they can come up against obstacles that allow them to struggle and cope and solve problems. Think of the increasing demands on families to meet external measures of success—starting academics earlier; rising amounts of homework and standardized testing; diminishing time for recess, physical education, creative arts, and music classes; overscheduling of after-school extracurriculars and tutoring; and so on. These are all activities meant to instill work ethic and goal-directedness in our children's growth trajectory. But when they crowd out adequate time for kids to be kids and explore their own interests in play, it can come with the significant cost of kids experiencing performance-driven anxiety at younger ages. In other words, not having enough time to develop the underlying structure that bolsters their ability to stay balanced, pay attention, and fully absorb new information can undermine children's academic success, and their future.

We want to therefore be careful not to overschedule our kids, or to prioritize their academic success at the expense of this other type of education, which is equally important *and also happens to keenly enable better academic performance.* After all, playfully engaging with our kids and allowing them to experience minor struggles and disappointments can enhance parts of their brains that help them approach obstacles—academic and otherwise—with flexibility and balanced thinking, rather than avoiding difficulties due to fear of failure and judgment.

> Not having enough time to develop the underlying structure that bolsters their ability to stay balanced, pay attention, and fully absorb new information can undermine children's academic success, and their future.

The second way we sometimes prevent kids from building more resilience has to do with how involved we become in their lives. *There's such a thing as too much scaffolding, just as it's possible to ask our kids to stretch beyond their capacity.* Sometimes we do too much; other times, we do not do enough. Do you fall on one side of the spectrum? Does it ever feel excruciating to watch your child solve a puzzle by themself or ride a scooter (even with helmet and kneepads) without your running along beside them? Do you ever find yourself taking the string cheese from your child's hands instead of allowing them to work through the difficulty of opening it themself? Tina admits to how hard this is for her with her boys and how she has to fight against this impulse every day, even as they move toward the end of adolescence. She still finds herself wanting to just take over, do things for them, rather than letting them work through what they need to do for themselves.

The same goes for Georgie. As the parent of a neurodivergent child, she doesn't always know how to gauge when he'll need her and when it's OK to let him try something on his own. When she's not sure, she challenges herself to wait a beat or two, often giving her nine-year-old son a few valuable seconds to process things and figure them out or to show where he still needs her. And the joy and surprise on his face when he can do it himself is priceless! But at times she feels tempted to step in too soon rather than letting him accomplish this small victory.

If you're like us, there's a good chance that your well-meaning intentions are getting in the way of your kids' opportunity to develop resilience, simply because you're not letting them work through a problem on their own. They're squarely in the ZPD, but instead of just offering support, you're taking over and thereby short-circuiting a process that would allow them to achieve mastery and develop confidence by facing and overcoming a challenging task or situation. That's too much *scaffolding*. When we lean too far in this direction, our kids can get the message that we don't think they can handle obstacles on their own, which can lead to a whole host of negative outcomes (like self-doubt, dependency, lower self-esteem, a tendency to listen too much to others' opinions, and so on).

On the other end of the continuum is the parent who doesn't step in *quite enough* when their child is struggling in the ZPD. Sometimes adults seem to believe that children should be able to complete a task that they're not yet developmentally capable of doing on their own. These parents withdraw or withhold their support at precisely the moment a child would greatly benefit from a sensitive, loving adult leaning closer to act as an emotional safety net—right when offering just enough support could allow the child to access a new ability or learn to tolerate a bit more frustration. That's too much *stretching*.

DO YOU EVER DEPRIVE YOUR CHILD OF RESILIENCE-BUILDING OPPORTUNITIES BY DENYING THEM THE CHANCE TO STRUGGLE?

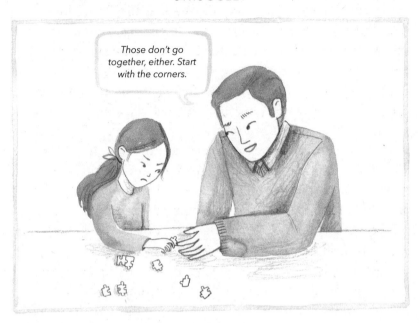

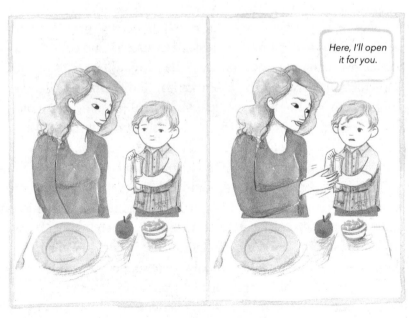

We've seen well-intentioned caregivers stand back with a kind of "How will they ever learn if I don't make them do it by themselves?" mentality as a child frantically sorts the parts of a science kit or throws an instruction manual on the floor, growing more despondent and lost without a caring helper available to assist in a pinch. It can be a deeply problematic worldview when adults hold the belief that children should face scary situations alone, or duke it out with the playground bully, or deal with academic problems in a dysregulated state without any support, simply because they believe it will toughen them up to survive in a difficult and unkind world.

> It can be a deeply problematic worldview when adults hold the belief that children should face scary situations alone, or duke it out with the playground bully, or deal with academic problems in a dysregulated state without any support, simply because they believe it will toughen them up to survive in a difficult and unkind world.

As we've said repeatedly in this book, we're all for providing boundaries and allowing children to face difficulties so they can learn to handle things for themselves. Kids need to be stretched. But we also encourage parents and teachers to be mindful of kids' individual and developmental differences as they consider how much challenge a child can manage at any given moment. Expecting young people to tackle excessive challenges alone may actually backfire in the long run, pushing a child too far beyond their abilities, leading them into patterns of dysregulated anger and reactivity or fear and fragility. Instead of achieving the resilience building we desire, kids may end up going in the opposite direction—avoiding challenges at any cost, shutting down, and withholding their true feelings from us—because they haven't received sensitively matched support within a predictable amount of safety.

DO YOU EVER DEPRIVE YOUR CHILD OF RESILIENCE-BUILDING OPPORTUNITIES BY WITHHOLDING SUPPORT BECAUSE YOU EXPECT TOO MUCH?

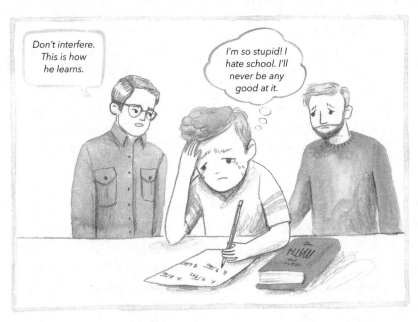

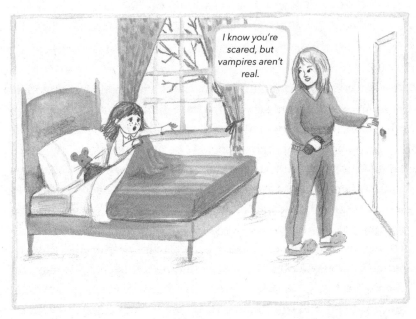

It's the classic Goldilocks conundrum. How do we offer the "just right" amount of scaffolding support so that we don't step in too much, yet also don't withhold the help our kids legitimately need? That's the focus of this fifth strategy, Scaffold and Stretch: using play to build grit and giving our kids opportunities to practice, in a supportive environment, the fundamental skills that culminate in a healthy and resilient mind.

Play as a Low-Stakes Road to Resilience

So when should real, authentic resilience building begin? Not when the risks are already very high. Instead, we want to foster the growth of crucial skills when stakes are low—when kids are just tinkering and participating in activities they enjoy—like playing.

You might think that play is all fun and games, affording children the luxury of already knowing exactly what they're doing and getting everything right the first time. Not so. As they explore in unstructured play, kids are constantly faced with their own limitations and repeatedly encounter difficulties that must be overcome. Their friend won't share or play the way they want them to. The beloved princess dress gets torn. Their battleship is sunk. The chute sends them right back to the beginning of the board game, just after they've climbed the long ladder. These valuable moments of frustration and annoyance come up time and again during play. Even in their own self-directed activity, children find that they can't control everything, so once again, play requires them to practice dealing with imperfection. Talk about learning to handle frustration!

In her studies looking at the speed at which children explore possible realities in their play, developmental scholar Alison Gopnik found that young children are rapid, sponge-like learners compared to adults. Adults take much longer pathways than kids do, even in solving relatively basic problems. In one study, Gopnik discovered that toddlers have greater mental flexibility, elasticity, and creativity than adults when facing challenges, and they're better at testing hypotheses. They do so intuitively through play. She illustrates this conclusion through an experiment where a box lights up if toy blocks are placed on it in a certain pattern. In one example, a child tests five hypotheses in a matter of minutes and efficiently figures it out. An adult then spends those minutes trying one hypothesis, and when it doesn't work, they sit there scratching their head. Children, as Gopnik shows, are naturally indefatigable problem solvers in play.

So if children are born to solve problems while they play, why bother teaching them to do so with more resilience? The reason is that we want to help them view their own mistakes and challenges through a positive lens, recognizing how valuable the difficult moments and the setbacks can be. Babies and toddlers don't at all mind making mistakes as they fumble with toys and bumble around; they're hardly conscious that anyone cares about doing things right. But around the time they head off to kindergarten, much of that changes for most kids. By that age, children have become shrewd observers, and they've begun to notice adults' nuanced and not-so-subtle emotional reactions to their flubs and errors. We get ruffled when they struggle to put on their shoes. We might knowingly and ironically smile at our partner or even cringe when our child sings off-key in the back seat. We're less happy when they miss a grounder at shortstop than we are when they make the play. Children learn, by watching us, that mistakes lead to feelings of worry, disappointment, and even shame. We're teaching them, in other words, that mistakes are bad and to be avoided.

If, on the other hand, we can work from the assumption that mistakes are valuable because they build resilience, then teach kids to see the world from that perspective, our children can get the message that errors don't necessarily detract from our enjoyment of the world. They can even be valuable. That's why we want to give them repeated practice dealing with small frustrations and learning the value of making mistakes, so that when bigger challenges come, they will have built skills at handling the tough stuff. And, if your child has a perfectionistic and anxious bend, it's even more important to give them opportunities to bounce back after setbacks.

Likewise, we want to model handling failures with levity and with an eye toward learning from setbacks. *I burned the bread again. Oh well. We'll cut off the edges and use extra butter. And now I know to set my timer for less time than the recipe suggests. Our oven is full of surprises!*

One of the other benefits of trying and failing is that it builds and hones executive functioning skills. As children leave behind the unfettered play of nursery school and adapt to structured learning, they'll need a robust set of executive functioning skills that will enable them to sit longer, focus better, and work smarter. Executive function is a highly complex set of skills that relies on many parts of the brain, including various parts of the cortex and midbrain. It serves to integrate and process complex information, direct attention where it needs to go, initiate tasks, manage time, shift gears when needed, regulate emotions, assess problems, adjust behavior, and more, accordingly. It allows children to do well in school and complete homework, chores, and other routine tasks. When kids' executive function skills are engaged, they can say confidently:

- I can focus my attention.
- I can visualize a plan.
- I can initiate and finish a task—even one I don't enjoy.
- I can remember the steps.
- I can filter out distractions.
- I can organize my materials.
- I can manage my time.
- I can redirect back if my attention gets snagged.
- I have tools to manage fear, frustration, or fatigue.
- I can monitor where I am, where I need to go, and what it's going to take to get me there.

It takes a long time, across the expanse of childhood as well as adolescence, for the parts of the brain that integrate these cognitive and emotional skills to fully mature and develop, and it takes lots of experimentation and practice over a stretch of years to strengthen those abilities.

And not to bum you out, but it may be as far away as the mid-to-late twenties that these skills are more automatic and robust! This sounds like bad news, but it's actually good because it means that we have a wide, long window during which our kids can gain the practice and the brain reps they need.

Virtually any parent of a college student or young adult will assure you that when your kid hits eighteen, as amazing as they are, you'll be starkly aware of how much development is still needed in the years to come. At that point you'll be relieved to know that the brain still has many more years ahead to keep maturing.

Kids, teens, and young adults need the freedom to figure some things out for themselves and try lots of different solutions as they work toward greater independence, and they should be allowed to experience plenty of penalty-free failures, as well as opportunities to learn from natural consequences. And a big part of our job is to provide connection and empathy when our children do have to face failures and negative ramifications of the choices they've made.

SOMETIMES WE NEED TO LET OUR KIDS DEAL WITH THE CONSEQUENCES OF THEIR DECISIONS. WE CAN STILL BE THERE FOR THEM WITHOUT "FIXING" THE PROBLEM.

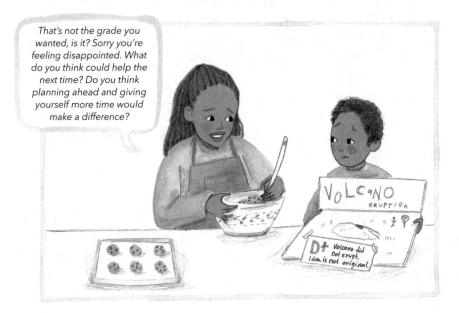

And yet, a vast majority of students as early as kindergarten are getting the message that they should be able to pull all these executive skills together with ease and coordinate tasks without making a mistake. So, not only are kids learning that there's something wrong with making mistakes, but they're also encountering unrealistic expectations of their executive functioning strategies too soon—at a time when these important skills, like initiating a performative task, working at it, and following through to achievement, should be cultivated instead through lots of exploration and trial and error.

When you two practice executing important tasks while you are playing, they can learn how to direct their attention, balance bigger emotions, and perform well under pressure, all in a setting where they know they can make mistakes without judgment. The stretching and scaffolding can take place at the same time. For kids who are neurodivergent, have ADHD, or are less mature in terms of their executive function, these strategies will be even more important in giving them the opportunities to build these skills as development unfolds.

Scaffold and Stretch: Step by Step

Let's talk about steps you can take as you play with your child that will offer both supportive scaffolding and opportunities to stretch. Each time you allow your child to face something difficult, while staying close by and offering help when truly needed, they have an opportunity to withstand negative emotions like frustration, disappointment, or a sense of failure, and come out feeling stronger for taking on adversity. Instead of rescuing or protecting them from challenges that would be good for them, we offer our presence enough to encourage their efforts, without taking over. Each successive attempt your child makes to expend effort toward a challenging task—with the tailored support they need from you so they can hang in there when it's really tough—broadens their skills so that their emotional regulation and executive function can work together.

As with the other strategies, Scaffold and Stretch involves a *simple* process that's not always *easy* to accomplish. Step 1, as you might guess by now, is to simply observe and attune to your child as you two begin to play.

Step 1: Observe your child, watching for signs they might benefit from a bit of support

We keep emphasizing this "observe and attune" step because so much of what we're teaching here begins with relationship and connection. If we aren't connected and tuned in to our children, then we're going to have a hard time knowing what they need in terms of their state of mind, and in terms of growth and skill building.

So begin by just keeping an eye on where things stand as you two begin to play. Watch closely and monitor for any stress signals. Is your child in the "regulated" section of the sensory dial? Even when things don't go as planned—the dog knocks over the tower, the eraser rips the paper, the plastic screwdriver head just *won't quite fit* into the screw—is your child able to keep trying or start anew if necessary? If so, and everything seems to be going well in terms of emotional balance and regulation, then there's likely not too much that you need to do in terms of offering assistance. Just enjoy being in the moment together and allow the time you're sharing to deepen and strengthen the bonds of your relationship.

Step 2: When necessary, offer scaffolding and stretching

When, however, your child begins to move toward more intense emotion (but not so far that they're losing control), that's when you know they're in the zone of proximal development—now's your chance to work with them to build grit and resilience. We spoke earlier about how some parents deny their kids resilience-building opportunities by not allowing them to struggle enough (too much scaffolding), while other parents make the mistake of not offering enough support when their children are having a hard time (too much stretching). A huge part of building resilience is about providing both scaffolding and stretching opportunities. And to know what's needed of each, you have to be attuned.

Sometimes Kids Are Ready to Be Stretched, Even When They Don't Know It

Kids often need our encouragement to keep going when they reach a place in their play where they become anxious, or they worry about taking the first (or the next) step. It might seem like a really small issue that doesn't make much sense to you: Maybe you and your kids are making play dough and your three-year-old won't participate because the mixture "looks yucky." Or perhaps you're teaching your seven-year-old to build a house of cards, but for some reason she shuts down, unwilling to add a card when it's her time. At other times your child's response might be more understandable—they lose a game against their uber-competitive brother and don't want to try another round, or they just don't feel comfortable taking another step toward the deep end of the pool to grab the ball you threw them.

Whether it's understandable to you or not, in all these cases it's probably time for you to step in and offer a gentle bit of scaffolding and support to help stretch your child so they can move back toward a state of mind that allows them to play without holding them back. You'd want to remain patient and supportive, obviously, but now's the time to encourage them to put a few fingers into the play-dough mix, or chance stacking the next card onto the house. They may need your help dealing with the gloating big brother, or with moving a few more inches toward deep water, so they can stay regulated and begin playing again.

Sometimes Kids Need More Support and Scaffolding

At other times, the last thing a kid needs is to be pushed to do more or try something they're not ready for. They might need to take incremental steps or they might need you to offer calm and support and to help them regulate their emotions and body so they can calm back

SOMETIMES YOUR CHILD IS READY TO BE STRETCHED, EVEN IF THEY DON'T REALIZE IT YET.

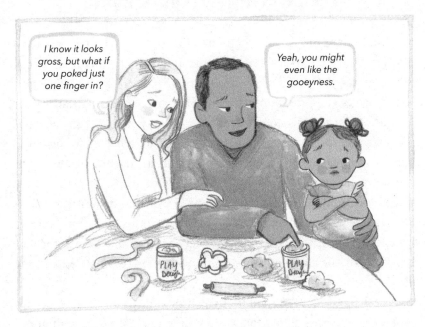

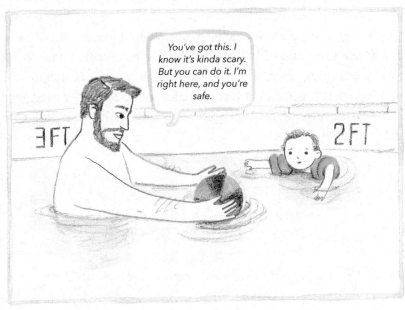

down. Here's an example of how one father, Jordan, found a way to offer scaffolding to his daughter, Macy, when she was tipping over into too much frustration and fear of failure as she was trying to complete her activities.

First, as Jordan observed and attuned, he noticed some telltale signs that Macy was running out of problem-solving grit and that her emotions were getting too intense. Did you know that kids can get mentally fatigued, even when they are "just playing"? It takes an enormous amount of physical and cognitive energy to keep pressing the gas and brakes on their nervous systems to keep directing attention where they want it to go. That's what Jordan noticed, that Macy was experiencing this depletion of energy and patience, so he checked in with his daughter. Their conversation went something like this:

Dad: Macy, you've been sitting in your play kitchen, fiddling with those apron strings, for a while. Everything OK? Need anything?

Macy: This stupid apron! I want to wear it, but I can't undo this knot! I hate it!

Dad: Oh, man, knots are hard sometimes! That drives me crazy, when I can't get one untied. And you've been working on this one a long time.

Macy: Here, you do it! (*Giving up, she throws the apron in his direction and turns her back to him, crying.*)

Dad: Oh, I see what you've been struggling with, sweetie. This is one of the tightest, most stubborn knots I've ever seen! Whoever tied this knot is an expert knot maker.

Macy: (*Wiping her tears*) It was me, Dad. I'm good at making knots, I just can't *undo* them. And I want to wear the apron now!

Dad: I hear you, sweetie. Let's look at it together. Hmmm. Where should we start? Which part of the knot should I pull on first? We can figure this out, no problem!

Notice how deftly Jordan swooped in, not to take over and fix the problem for his daughter but to allow her to first experience her frustration in his calm presence. She didn't need to be stretched right then—she was already working hard to solve the problem. She just couldn't, at least on her own, get that "stupid" knot untied. What she needed was the scaffolding support that could help her calm down some, so that she and her dad could work together on the apron strings. She was frustrated but not dysregulated yet. His response allowed her to stay regulated enough to learn, stretch her frustration tolerance, push through, and problem-solve. She was right in the ZPD, fully primed to grow from the experience if her dad handled things well. And fortunately, he did. There are going to be times when our children simply can't complete a difficult activity without an adult's help— maybe it's beyond their age or developmental level or they are too fatigued in the moment—and that's perfectly OK. Our focus should be on giving them the cushion to make that transition from feeling irritated, incompetent, and overwhelmed to regaining composure, so they can accomplish the task and move toward mastery. At times, providing the cushion might mean noticing when they become dysregulated and flooded with intense emotion, in which case you can go back to supporting them with co-regulation, helping their nervous systems get regulated again so they can return to play and exploration.

SOMETIMES YOUR CHILD NEEDS SOME
SCAFFOLDING AND SUPPORT.

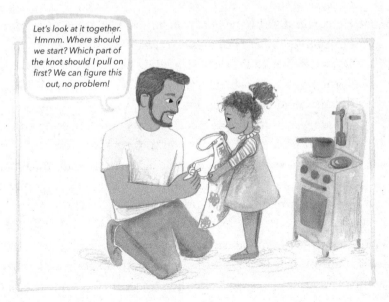

Scaffolding as an Assistant

When you notice frustration building in your child, and you see the potential that they might blow up over frustrating tasks—like when they can't pull two Lego bricks apart, or unzip the veterinarian's bag, or make a picture look perfect—one of the best ways to provide support is to step in and offer to be your child's assistant.

Notice that when Macy needed help, Jordan didn't just step in and take the reins. In certain situations you may need to do that, but when possible, it's better to allow your child to maintain agency and autonomy over the situation at hand.

Sure, they may cry out, "I can't do this! You do it for me!" Those are their big feelings talking. But really, it's more likely the case that they actually *can* do it; they just need some help. They might simply need you to guide their attention to the smallest first step that needs to be taken. Or they might need broader directions than that.

Either way, having you step in to simply assist, *while allowing your child to gain the benefits of continuing to work through the problem,* can help them continue building grit and resilience. And it works wonders, in terms of helping them return to a place of emotional regulation, if you are the one holding the knotted apron strings, or the dried glue bottle, or the zipper on the veterinarian's kit bag. It can provide significant relief from some of their distress to see the source of their discomfort being *literally* held in the capable hands of their caring assistant. That's supportive scaffolding.

Seeing the problem in someone else's hands can often calm your child enough to move them out of the overwhelm zone and into the ZPD. And that's one of the best places they can be, if we want them to build more resilience. Once your child trusts that you're able to assist them in handling the problem, and they realize that they don't have to know everything or solve it all by themself, you can use a reassuring tone as you hold up the item so they can look at it with greater control and perspective. Questions like, "Hmm. Where should we start?" or "How do you think we should fix this thing?" can stimulate their attention and problem-solving ability, as if you're simply a novice who needs their expert opinion.

ACTING AS YOUR CHILD'S ASSISTANT CAN HELP MOVE THEM
BACK INTO EMOTIONAL REGULATION.

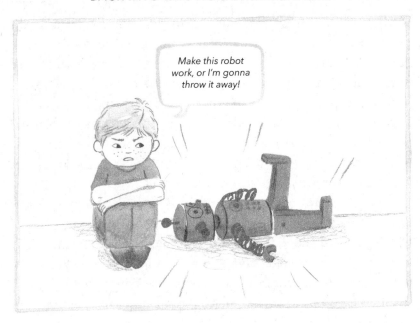

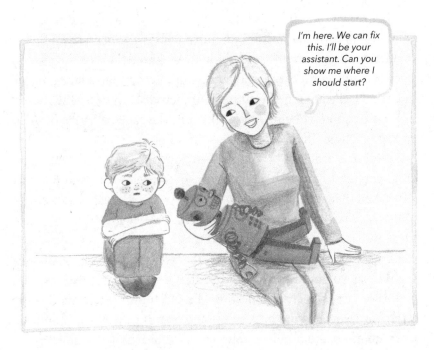

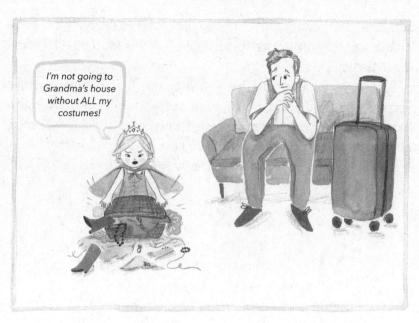

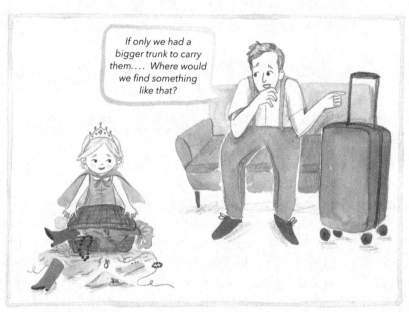

At the same time, you fully intend to utilize their guidance and coaching to resolve the issue, thereby reengaging and expanding their executive skills and ability to keep trying. Ultimately, if they're thinking hard enough and communicating well enough to coach someone else to do it, then those higher parts of the brain are back online, and they're once again capable of learning from this challenging experience.

Again, we're not saying that you shouldn't hold boundaries that keep objects from being destroyed or people from being hurt; some behaviors may need to be addressed once your child has calmed down. The point here is about ways you can get them calm that much more quickly, helping them move toward mastering a difficult situation.

> We're not saying that you shouldn't hold boundaries that keep objects from being destroyed or people from being hurt; some behaviors may need to be addressed once your child has calmed down. The point here is about ways you can get them calm that much more quickly, helping them move toward mastering a difficult situation.

Often, resilience grows exponentially if we shine a spotlight on a solution, without telling kids exactly how to do it, because they believe they found the answer on their own. Even if we provide additional support, hints, and suggestions the whole way along, children are much more likely to remember the end of an experience rather than how it began. So although things might have gotten off to a rough start, helping a child find their own solution and finish strong is the real magic of developing grit. When kids struggle but believe they've found the answer and completed the challenging task for themselves, they often feel a huge rush of dopamine, the intrinsic reward hormone that reinforces a behavior, and the sweet triumph of their own success. Then, that resilience can snowball into higher self-esteem and a greater ability to persevere and think of better solutions the next time.

A TINY BIT OF RESILIENCE CAN SNOWBALL OVER TIME.

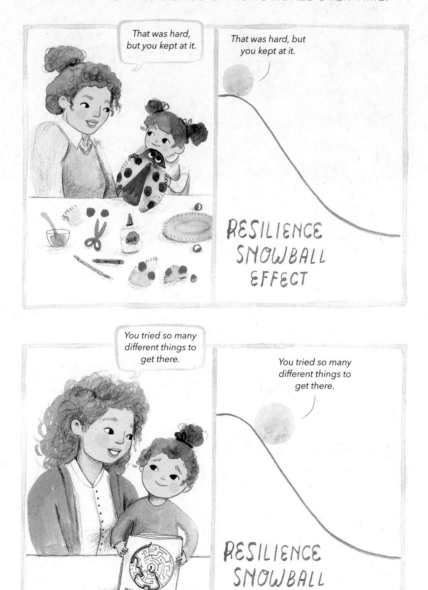

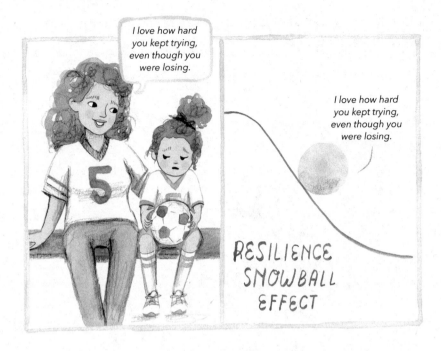

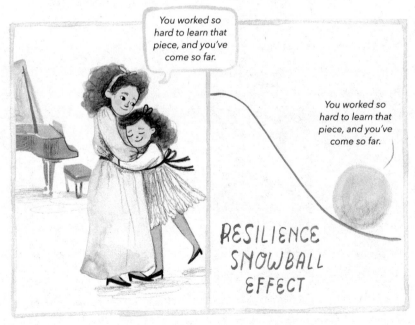

A Final Case Study

Before we close, let us tell you about a boy who Georgie worked with in her play therapy practice. We'll call him Alfie, and his mom and dad were worried that he tended to fall apart emotionally anytime a challenge appeared. Even a minor hiccup could cause him emotional strife: He'd fly into a rage when he couldn't find the right color of cape for his action figure, or he'd fall on the floor in despair because two Tinker Toys wouldn't fit correctly, no matter how hard he tried to cram them together.

If any of this sounds familiar, and you've noticed a similar tendency in your own child when daily tasks or activities become challenging, you might be relieved to hear that many children are still working on tethering their emotional skills to their executive abilities, and this can lead to extremely strong emotional reactions around the slightest sign of difficulty. In Alfie's case, he was still learning how to tether his attention ("I can stay focused and remember the steps") to his emotional regulation ("I have tools to manage fear and frustration").

A helpful and effective approach for building executive and emotional skills for children like Alfie, who skyrocket into big emotions and angrily melt down when they perceive obstacles, is to scaffold in the underlying skills they need when they're playing in a more regulated state, while they can still think calmly and solve problems. This is what Georgie did with Alfie while he was playing with some action figures in her office. She got to do some proactive resilience building while he was in the ZPD.

Everything seemed fine to start with. Alfie was directing the figures with simple actions, like having them walk around, put on their armor, and scuffle with some bad guys. He was happily cruising along without a problem in sight, until he decided the action men should load their gear into some sort of vehicle so they could get to the next battle. That's when things started to get heated. Alfie tended to feel stressed when he couldn't instantly find a suitable car or truck, so Georgie stayed close beside him and described the steps he was taking on the search. She said things like, "Looks like that car's too small.

Hmm, so is the pickup. But you're still looking." (Remember Think Out Loud, the first PlayStrong strategy?)

Because Georgie saw that he was not enjoying his increasingly chaotic experience—the lack of control, more fear and uncertainty about finding the desired transport vehicle, the possibility of failure and disappointment—she knew that she needed to act as his assistant and scaffold his efforts by "lending" him her prefrontal executive functions. She kept using the Think Out Loud strategy and simply described the steps she saw him taking to help him stay focused on the task. That way, as frustration began to arise, he could borrow those executive skills from an emotionally regulated adult as he dealt with the unpleasant feelings, the aggravation, and the swirls of fear, as he continued his search. In so doing, she helped stack several skills Alfie could practice simultaneously, as he successfully held his emotions in check and stayed focused on the task, building the upper and lower parts of the brain that give rise to more resilient kids. Her scaffolding allowed him to stretch. He got to practice tolerating frustration enough to keep going and move toward problem-solving instead of a meltdown.

Along the way, Georgie kept observing and attuning, watching closely and monitoring for stress signals that would warn her that Alfie might be starting to "lose it" or get dangerously close to becoming too intense. That would cue her that more emotional support—more scaffolding—might be needed. Luckily, Alfie spotted a big yellow school bus that would fit the action figures and their armor and other gear, resulting in a whoop for joy, as the boy's rewarding feelings (and the accompanying surge of happy hormones like dopamine and serotonin) counteracted the stress and gave a significant boost to the grit he gained from the experience.

But bigger problems were yet to come that would test Alfie's grit and further stretch him. He soon discovered that he didn't know how to get the action figures into the bus. They wouldn't fit through the main entrance. Georgie noticed that he was clenching his teeth, and he began to stomp the feet of the soldier he was holding, all the while narrowing his eyes at the door of the bus. All signs pointed to the possibility that he was at the very edge of the ZPD and moving perilously close to entering the overwhelm zone. Could Georgie keep him holding on long enough in the ZPD to increase his sense of resilience and grit?

She looked for ways she could be his assistant and offer small increments of well-timed support, with hints that would keep him trying, focused, and not giving up. Here's how the conversation went:

Alfie: (*frustrated, trying to cram the figures through the bus's door*) They won't go in!

Georgie: (*with some enthusiasm and purpose, almost like a coach*) OK, Alfie, I'm right here with you. We can do this together. You know this bus better than I do. Is there any way besides the main door?

Alfie: There's a button on the roof! I'll press that . . .

Georgie: Great discovery! Hmm, that turned on the headlights. You're still working hard to get these guys on the bus.

Alfie: But that didn't work. I'll squeeze this smaller guy through the window.

Georgie: You're coming up with lots of ideas, and you're not giving up.

Alfie: Argh, he doesn't fit!

Georgie: You've really narrowed it down. We know what's not working. But it looks like there's still one more opening you haven't tried . . .

Alfie: Hang on, there's a back door! Like on a real school bus!

Georgie: You got it, Alfie! Because you kept trying. That must feel amazing!

Yes, Georgie is a professional play therapist. But notice that she didn't do anything here that you couldn't do with your own kids. She simply observed and attuned, then watched for opportunities to both scaffold and stretch. She avoided taking over and instead loaned Alfie her executive skills by serving as his assistant. And as a result, he was able to work through some obstacles that might otherwise have upset him pretty quickly.

Each time you help your children get to the other side of an obstacle like this, you give them a little bit more grit. When kids have lots of small grit-building experiences, they collect and accumulate them as a framework for feeling more self-confident and competent to take on positive risks and more challenging situations. In other words, that confidence and competence become part of their working model for interacting with their world.

> Each time you help your children get to the other side of an obstacle, you give them a little bit more grit. When kids have lots of small grit-building experiences, they collect and accumulate them as a framework for feeling more self-confident and competent to take on positive risks and more challenging situations. In other words, that confidence and competence become part of their working model for interacting with their world.

These minor wins get stored up and remembered along neural pathways that can be reactivated and applied to major life challenges your child will face as they grow up, becoming more resilient each time they overcome an impediment. "I can work hard under pressure." "I can keep going even when I'm worried about failure." "Mistakes are an important path to learning." "I believe in myself enough to try again." Declarations like these get practiced again and again, becoming not just affirming statements to say to themselves in the mirror but enduring internal belief systems that will pay huge dividends to their sense of self when dealing with adverse experiences, both now and in the future.

STRATEGY **# 6 :**

Narrate to Integrate

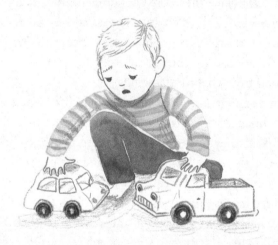

Primary skill being developed in the child:
Use of stories to better comprehend and deal with difficult
circumstances.

Primary message received by the child:
Stories can help me understand what's going on around me, so I can
make better choices.

In the aftermath of the September 11 terrorist attacks in New York City, many children exhibited trauma symptoms such as trouble sleeping, worry and agitation, fears about the safety of their loved ones, a desire to stay home from school, difficulty concentrating, and even regression in skills they had already mastered. Feelings of hopelessness also showed up in their play, a major indicator that they had gone through an enormously difficult event that temporarily stressed or halted development and put them in survival mode.

Play therapists were some of the first invited to tend to children's emotional needs post-9/11, and what they noticed was that the kids were replaying scenes of loss—in their minds and talking about them, too—without any hope of resolution. Without an outlet for expressing what they had been through, these children had no way of getting beyond the horrifying images, sounds, and smells they'd witnessed. The clinicians therefore encouraged the kids to use play, art, music, and other forms of creative expression to unlock and process their trauma and grief. Throughout the process, the therapists again and again witnessed the power of story to help the children work through their overwhelming feelings.

What the clinicians repeatedly found is that when children are faced with unspeakable events where they can't find the words to express all that they're feeling, storytelling can become a powerful coping mechanism. It allows kids to locate the problem and use any means at their disposal to create more hopeful solutions, even if they must tap into fantasy to dream up resolutions that couldn't exist in reality (like helpful dinosaurs working alongside other heroes in one case). A child's healthy urge to solve problems is so powerful that the kids were able to move through unimaginable loss, pain, and fear by imagining solutions that could exist only in their minds. In doing so, they found more comfort and avoided further trauma and anxiety when they pictured the helpers and imagined what it would be like to rebuild. Almost instinctively, the kids used narrative to get back on track with development and move toward post-traumatic recovery and growth.

You can give your children similar tools and strategies to use with either large-T Traumas (like a national tragedy or the death of a loved one) or small-t traumas (like conflict with siblings and friends or a trip to the dentist). Storytelling is a powerful strategy in all kinds of other situations, too—not only when it comes to dealing with difficult moments and memories. When you allow and encourage your kids to tell stories as they play, you offer the potential for imagination, emotion, and creativity to ignite the flames of wonder in their young minds. You provide the possibility for cognitive, social, and emotional development. And you introduce them to powerful tools for solving problems and handling conflict in a metaphorical place that's safe enough for them to work through and get clear on what's going on inside themselves. These are the goals and desired outcomes of the next PlayStrong strategy, Narrate to Integrate.

Storytelling can help you better understand your child and assist them in developing a stronger personal and moral compass so they can navigate their inner and outer emotional lives with less struggle and more well-being.

The Power of Story

Let's look at specific ways stories can offer powerful support in a child's development. This list could go on and on, so we'll focus on only a few of the most beneficial ways you can use narrative to encourage your kids and help them grow.

Stories help kids solve problems faster and with more resilience

One of the most important uses of storytelling in play is related to the one we've primarily focused on so far in this chapter: It helps kids figure out how to deal with tricky and potentially upsetting problems. Stories aren't always nice, but they are necessary. Children introduce difficulties in their made-up stories that may often closely resemble real-life challenges and conflicts that they haven't fully figured out yet.

> S tories aren't always nice, but they are
> necessary.

What's more, stories help kids rapidly test out many solutions in play and consider different outcomes that enhance their problem-solving ability, especially as they're learning to balance how to solve the problem (which requires the logic of the left brain) with the worry or frustration about finding the best solution (part of the job of the right brain).

One child might create a play scene that contains a moral conundrum that they are trying to think through—maybe a character wants to swipe a cookie from the jar but knows he should ask first. Another child might need to sort through mixed-up feelings about a problem or conflict—possibly playing out how she could deal with an aggressive schoolmate who also happens to be a close friend.

Stories offer children what play therapists call "symbolic distance," which means that kids can explore sensitive topics more easily in their play because it's "not real, just pretend," where they feel the emotions connected to the experience with less intensity and where strife and overwhelm can be safely contained. This symbolic distance lets kids explore themes that feel too big and overwhelming, or that are too abstract to make complete sense of at their age and cognitive level.

They learn to handle conflicts, both external and internal. They can use the safety of metaphors in imaginary play to represent and reenact conflicts they've had with other people, and to do so free of stress or consequences as they try different solutions until one of them works. Or they can take an internal conflict or problem they've been wrestling with, something they wouldn't even be able to articulate in words very well, and express it in ways that can be seen, sorted, and solved better in fantasy than reality.

PLAYFUL STORYTELLING HELPS KIDS
THINK THROUGH STICKY SITUATIONS.

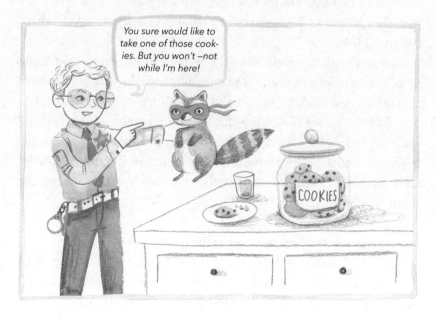

Stories help kids develop empathy

The world is a complicated place, and as children grow up, we need to help them learn to negotiate it in all its complexity. That means teaching them to move beyond oversimplification and egocentrism. Some of childhood's most common go-to responses to conflict—tattling, fighting back, insisting on their preference, getting even—are based on an assumption that there's only one way to look at a situation: our own.

So we need to help our kids move beyond this one-sided perspective and recognize a story's inherent complexity, consider another's perspective, work to resolve disagreements, take responsibility for their part of the conflict, and become proactive in being part of the solution. These skills are evidence that kids are gaining greater insight, perspective, and maturity, all of which are necessary to live a life full of meaning, significance, and relational well-being.

Really, what we're talking about here is a value we've discussed several times already in the book: empathy. When we can approach the world with empathy, we'll be able to feel with others and avoid assuming that our perspective is the only one that matters. And when kids tell stories that ask them to get into the minds of their characters, they necessarily improve their ability to imagine what others feel and think.

That means that, later, when they're in an actual, real-world argument with a sibling or a soccer teammate, they'll be that much better at listening and working to come to a solution that honors both parties. By helping them develop this crucial relational skill, you'll be ensuring that as they get older, they'll enjoy deeper and more meaningful relationships—with their family, their friends, and eventually their romantic partners. Ultimately, that's what we're aiming for when we narrate to integrate.

Stories help kids share their inner life

As we've said, children show us a great deal about what's going on in their minds when they tell stories. If we simply pay attention, we'll hear about what they fear, love, worry about, and hope for.

PLAYFUL STORYTELLING TELLS YOU WHAT KIDS:

FEAR.

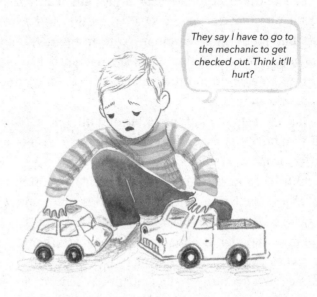

They say I have to go to the mechanic to get checked out. Think it'll hurt?

LOVE.

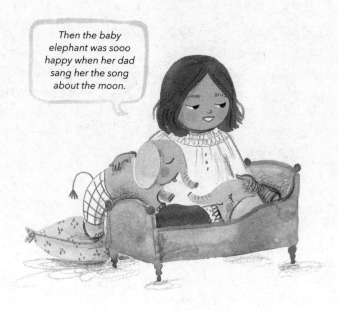

WORRY ABOUT.

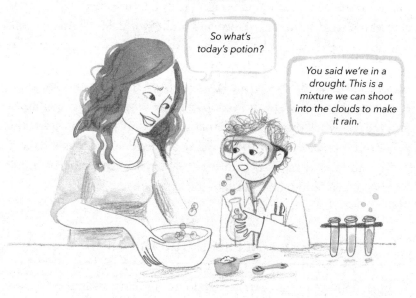

HOPE FOR.

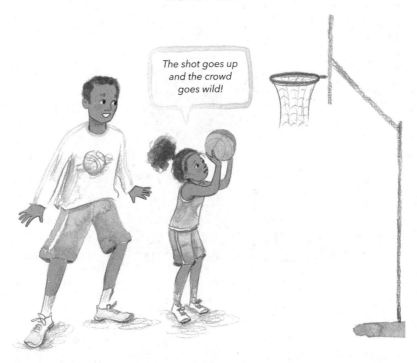

Storytelling is so natural and omnipresent in the lives of children that we often underestimate its significance. Stories help kids gather new knowledge, understand the ways of the world, and figure out the solutions to tricky problems. It can also be great for parents, who reap lots of rewards when they raise an avid storyteller who remembers details and enjoys sharing specifics from their life and imagination. Whether you want the scoop on how a fight between siblings erupted, or what kind of problematic situations popped up on the playground or in the classroom, many of the typical issues kids face can be addressed more expeditiously when you hear their unique perspective on and recollection of the experience.

The Story Arc: Dig into the Middle

Almost 2,500 years ago, Aristotle told his audiences something they probably already knew and that we all know today: A story should have a beginning, a middle, and an end. It's what we call the classic story arc, and it's likely what you see in the narratives your children tell as well. Maybe they're building on classic tales like "Jack and the Beanstalk" or "Goldilocks and the Three Bears," or they might be aiming for something more like what they see in the Star Wars or Marvel universe. Or maybe they're making up an entirely new narrative of their own. Regardless of how iconic, archetypal, cultural, or original the story is, and whether your kids are using action figures, puppets, costumes, or props such as a doctor kit or kitchen set, they're probably following the classic story arc: Action and conflict appear and then rise toward a climax, after which we see some sort of resolution. Along the way, characters usually learn valuable lessons that make them smarter, more agile in problem-solving, and wiser about how the world works.

THE CLASSIC STORY ARC.

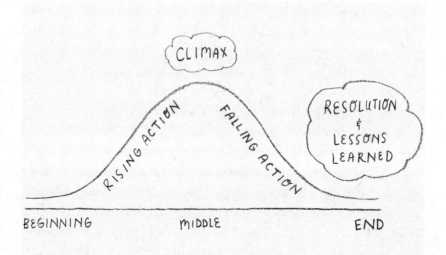

As we listen to our kids' stories, we want to watch for how they introduce the narrative. What's the setting? A deep, dark forest? In space? At the hospital? Also, what's the situation? Is there a bank robbery? Is someone late for a concert? And who are the characters? Mommy and baby? The farm animals? Beyoncé and Jay-Z? These details make up a story's *beginning*.

Once the stage has been set, children fairly quickly introduce the idea that there's trouble afoot, or an inciting incident takes place. Perhaps the latch to the lion's cage was not properly closed and the giant animal is now on the loose, so the story escalates with rising action as the zookeepers scramble to find the lion before it gobbles up all the flamingos. Here we witness the rise of growing conflict. Who left the latch undone? Can they protect the flamingos? Will the zookeepers work as a good team, or will they bumble around, make too many mistakes, and get gobbled up, too? Will one zookeeper emerge as the confident and capable hero?

This section of a narrative is what we call the *middle,* and it's the place that we suggest parents really dig into the story, as kids build to a dramatic turning point in the narrative. The reason is that the middle typically affords the most opportunities for exploring how to resolve internal emotional struggles and conflicts between characters as the story then moves toward a resilience-building ending. Children take great delight in devising the engagements themselves, not just to entertain themselves but so they can be the ones to solve the problem, developing their own tools of conflict resolution. So that's where you want to focus your attention: on this middle phase of the story arc, where you can get more clear on the conflict at play, then help them reframe it if necessary. (We'll discuss this idea soon.)

As the story moves toward a resolution and reaches its end, you have the opportunity to elevate the bigger meaning, or theme, of the story, allowing your child to remember important life lessons or takeaway messages from the storytelling experience. The point isn't at all that you make every narrative a fable that concludes with a "the moral of the story is" type of ending. That would strip all the pleasure from the narrative. But still, you can add little details to a story that take it to a new level in terms of meaning and significance.

Again, you don't have to make every aspect of playtime "educational." In fact, please don't! Kids will hate that. It's educational all on its own, and if you're heavy-handed with making it didactic, it takes away the fun. This makes kids want to do it less, which means they'll learn less!

But as you play, and as you and your child enjoy the various stories involved in the process, watch for subtle ways to prioritize and emphasize principles and perspectives that you'd like for your child to internalize.

SOMETIMES YOU CAN REFRAME THE CONFLICT TO HELP YOUR CHILD GAIN A NEW PERSPECTIVE.

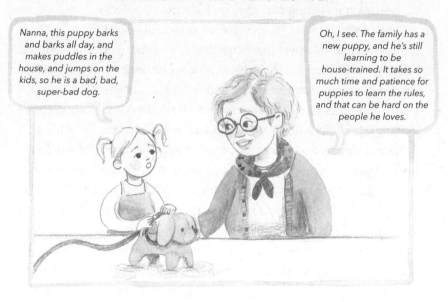

WATCH FOR WAYS TO ELEVATE THE MEANING OF A STORY.

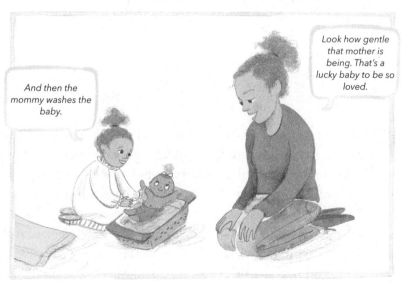

Horizontal Integration: Working from Both Sides of the Brain

Before we get to the step-by-step process involved in narrating to integrate, it's important to understand a concept that will increase the impact storytelling can have on kids' development.

One of the reasons stories are so powerful—for kids as well as adults—is that they perform extremely important work in the brain. Namely, they allow for the critical process of horizontal *integration*. This mechanism is multifaceted and complex, but the basic concept is fairly simple and easy to understand. (If you know Tina's book with Dan Siegel, *The Whole-Brain Child*, you're already familiar with it.)

Neural integration takes place when separate parts of the brain work together as a whole. For example, in past chapters we've been discussing top-down and bottom-up parental approaches. That's an example of *vertical* integration, where the higher and lower parts of the brain are encouraged to work together. *Horizontal* neural integration, then, takes place when the left and right hemispheres of the brain work together to do what neither could accomplish on its own.

> Horizontal neural integration takes place when the left and right hemispheres of the brain work together to do what neither could accomplish on its own.

We're going to oversimplify here a bit, but the basic idea is one that many people are already familiar with: that we can think of the two sides of the brain performing different types of mental processing. What we'll call left-brain processing allows for our thinking that's often characterized as logical, analytical, language-based, and detail-oriented. The right brain, on the other hand, is typically linked with intuition, creativity, and more holistic or contextualized thinking. It helps with tasks like artistic expression, pattern recognition, bodily control, and emotional awareness. And whereas the left brain loves words and structure, the right brain is nonverbal.

Again, the actual processes in the different parts of the brain are much more complicated than what we're describing here, but this perspective helps us understand important attributes of how our brain processes information. When we think of the different tendencies of what we're calling the left and right brain, we can begin to see why horizontal integration would be so powerful—it combines the left-brain logic and language skills with the right-brain emotion and contextual thinking, allowing a person to approach a situation from a much fuller perspective.

There's probably no better place to witness that process and the power of integration than in storytelling. Think of a time your three-year-old got hurt. Maybe he hit his head while crawling under the kitchen table. In that moment, he's flooded with pain, along with shock and fear from his right brain. As adults, when we hit our head or bang our knee on something, we experience the pain, but we have enough life experience to realize that the pain will soon subside. A young child, though, knows only that he's hurting, and as far as he knows he might be in pain forever. What he needs in that moment, then, is for you to step in and bring some integration to the situation, adding left-brain logic. He needs your words and your logical explanation to help him understand what happened and what he's currently experiencing.

How do you do that? With a story. You talk him through his experience, using your words to bring some order to what just happened. You narrate to integrate. "You were crawling under the table, and BUMP! you hit your head right here." You might even act it out for him, helping him visualize the scene. (This would be a great time for gentle humor and playfulness, by the way.) In this moment, as he watches your reenactment, there's a good chance that he'll stop crying, fascinated by the narrative you're spinning.

As you continue *narrating*, you'll be *integrating* the left and right, helping your child deal with his experience by bringing in the more rational part of the brain to work in concert with the emotional. That's the power of story. And that's the power you can harness when your child tells stories while you two are playing together.

STORIES HELP INTEGRATE THE BRAIN.

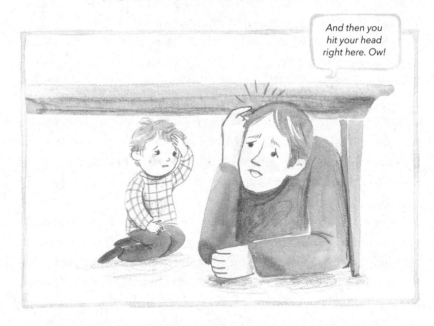

Narrate to Integrate: Step by Step

As always, you want to begin by paying close attention to what you're seeing and hearing from your children as they tell their stories. Once again, your first step is to observe and attune. After that: oscillate, integrate, and elevate. Let's break it down.

Step 1: Observe and attune

Stories that kids tell—and actually, this applies to adults as well—often disclose more than the narrator consciously realizes. One reason is that sometimes the spotlight of left-brained awareness hasn't been turned on just yet. Stories are typically full of right-brain details where our mind is mapping our feelings and sensations, or the nonverbal content of our lived experiences. These all get stored in memory and can be expressed in play (and other modes of communication).

Both good and bad experiences are encoded as embodied implicit memories that can therefore be difficult to access, and hard to describe in words, depending on the nature of the experience. Verbally and reasonably expressing ourselves about problems and conflicts is hard even for adults, and it's harder still for kids, especially when tensions are high or they're processing a difficult or painful memory. When children feel overwhelmed by conflicts in the real world, we often see themes of those unresolved situations coming out in right-brained play.

For example, a common occurrence is that a young child with a new sibling plays with a baby doll. She might initially act out a story where she's feeding and changing the doll, but then begins to bop the doll on the head and complain that "the baby is always crying." Or a child who's struggling after recently changing schools might act out scenes with mean kids, overly strict rules, or a ridiculous amount of classroom discipline issues.

So when our child is telling a story, we need to tune in and watch for what's going on beyond the obvious, surface-oriented plot of the narrative. That's when we can put our knowledge about horizontal integration to work.

An important note: We're focusing here primarily on stories where children are to some extent working through questions or struggles that might be at work within them, often without their knowledge. That means that we'll be discussing the importance of paying attention to what might be taking place *beyond and beneath* the more obvious plot points of a story.

But we want to make it clear that sometimes a story is just a story. In other words, children often simply become caught up in creating a narrative that's fun or exciting or dangerous or dramatic or something else. In those cases, they're not subconsciously working through problems or trying to understand something more fully on a subliminal level. They might just be trying on what it feels like to act out different roles and express different traits and emotions. So don't put pressure on yourself to mine each narrative interaction with your child for some sort of subconscious meaning or import. Much of the time, you can just enjoy the plot and interact in ways that foster that joy and exuberance for narrative your child is experiencing.

Sometimes, though, there might be more than meets the eye in what your child is giving attention to, and that's when you want to watch for ways to bring in the horizontal integration that can work real magic in the interaction, and in your child's development. This type of integration can help defuse automatic resistance when you're asking your child to clean up or switch off a screen or device. It can offer alternatives to more reactive responses to conflict with siblings or classmates. It can address areas that seem to provoke a child to be oversensitive. And it can replace certain familiar go-to defense mechanisms like arguing, blaming, or complaining.

When you help bring integration into a story and into the surrounding situation, you enable kids to learn new ways of dealing with conflict, and you create the circumstances for replacing old patterns of automatic and suboptimal responses to real-life struggles.

Step 2: Oscillate

The second step is all about emphasizing both the right and left processing as you interact with your child while they're telling a story. If you can oscillate back and forth between the right and the left, you'll begin to move your child toward an integrated state where they can use more than just one part of their brain.

> If you can oscillate back and forth between the right and the left, you'll begin to move your child toward an integrated state where they can use more than just one part of their brain.

Again, the right-brain details are usually already present in a child's narrative, especially if something's bothering them. But kids don't always tell clear, easy-to-follow stories, and that fact can make it challenging for us as parents. When children aren't operating from a state of integrated play, they're less likely to offer an organized, logical, linear series of events. In some cases, kids might share facts about the story, but we don't see how those pieces tie together to create an overarching meaning, a big picture of why the story holds together or matters. Or their stories may be so full of drama and intense emotions, with lots of madcap cartoon antics or slapstick humor intended to amuse their play partner, that they come across as too chaotic to follow or lacking in substance.

What kids often need, then, is for adults to help invite the left hemisphere into the conversation, so it can look over the details of the experience and add verbal descriptions, creating more of an orderly sequence of events. Especially when a story is clouded by intense imagery around problems and difficulties, it can be hard to find the logic in why these events are taking place—sometimes we can't even tell for sure that it's a story at all. You know it's time to bring in some left-brain thinking when narrative details aren't in linear order or when a child is struggling to find the language to describe what's happening. In these cases, it can be almost impossible to find a resolution to the story's conflict because it's so disorganized.

That's when we need to step in and help out, either by asking clarifying questions or by making suggestions that can help elucidate where the story is going. Your task isn't to take over the narrative process—you definitely want to allow your child to maintain ownership of and authority over the story they're telling—but they might need some nudging that can allow them to make things clear enough to understand.

But your job's not complete just because you've begun to offer some narrative order. After bringing in the logic from the left, watch to further develop the more right-brained aspects of the story again. Remember, the right-brain mode of processing allows for understanding the whole context of a situation and pulling out the bigger meaning of our experiences. It helps create what psychologists call autobiographical meaning, which lets us figure out "what this means for who I am." So that's what we do after we've

SOMETIMES KIDS NEED YOU
TO HELP BRING SOME LEFT-BRAIN LOGIC TO THEIR STORIES.

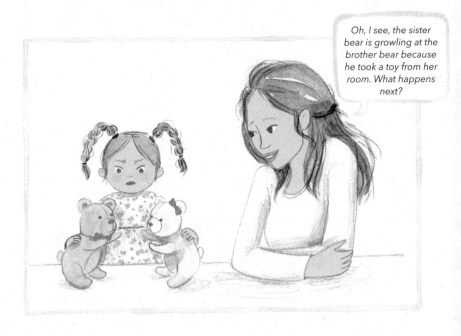

Oh, I see, the sister bear is growling at the brother bear because he took a toy from her room. What happens next?

helped our child bring in the structure and verbal order to discover new solutions to the current problem: We oscillate back to the right, moving to a place where they can create new experiences to replace the older feelings, viewing deeper themes and meanings that let them see the situation from a broader perspective. That's how we narrate to integrate.

Then, most likely, you'll see a need at some point to move to the left again, then possibly back to the right. The idea is that we remain flexible and nimble as we play with our child and listen to their stories, ready to horizontally oscillate back and forth. We can connect with the right by getting clear on the problem as the child feels and experiences it, then move into the left brain by helping clarify the issues at hand, then bring in context with the right, then look for solutions together until the child can find the best one, then return to discuss resulting emotions and perceptions based on what the child sees. And on and on—rinse and repeat. As the focus oscillates

AFTER INTRODUCING LOGIC, INJECT SOME RIGHT-BRAIN
CONTEXTUAL THINKING TO HELP CREATE NEW SELF-
UNDERSTANDING AND AUTOBIOGRAPHICAL MEMORY.

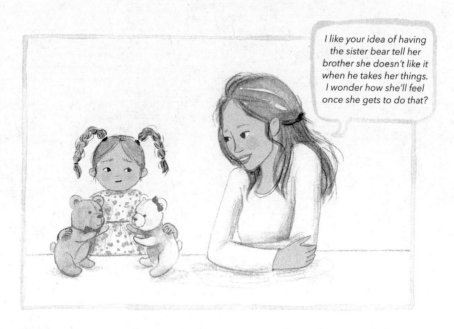

between left and right, you'll be narrating to integrate, and your child
will be getting practice at using both modes of processing.

Step 3: Integrate and elevate

Once we've moved back and forth, oscillating between left and right
modes of processing, the integration process will begin to occur
fairly naturally. Deeper themes in stories can form new explicit
memories that can be discussed, explained, and understood by others, with a stronger, more coherent sense of self-efficacy and self-
direction. The point, in other words, is to *integrate* left and right, so
you can then *elevate* the bigger meaning of the story, bringing in
important life lessons or takeaway messages from the storytelling
experience.

For example, imagine that your fourth grader and her friend enlist
you to be the customer in their pretend restaurant. Without being

WATCH FOR WAYS TO INTEGRATE AND ELEVATE.

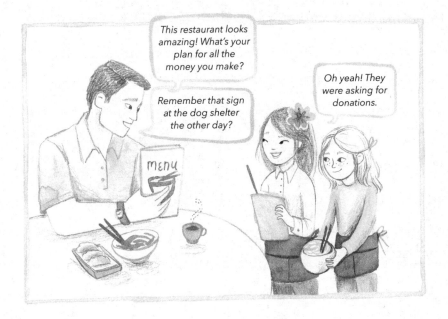

preachy or taking the fun out of the game, is there a way you can ask a question about making good decisions with the money we earn from our jobs?

Notice that this dad used logic while also appealing to his daughter's emotions and morals. This integrative approach simultaneously engaged different parts of her brain and challenged her to add something bigger, something deeper, to the story she and her friend were acting out.

That might seem easier to do with older kids, but younger children's stories offer the same opportunity. Narrating to integrate doesn't even have to be a lesson with huge moral or ethical implications. You can use stories to integrate and elevate in ways that send messages your child needs to hear—like when he's worried about his first day of kindergarten. Maybe he's into astronomy, and the night before the first day of school, you tell a story that involves becoming a famous scientist. Then you can tag on a detail that elevates the story into something he can carry with him the next day when he feels anxious.

WATCH FOR WAYS TO INTEGRATE AND ELEVATE.

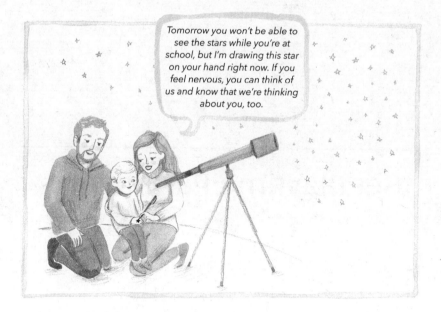

The point is that you're finding ways to maintain the fun of storytelling—that's crucial—while also appealing to different parts of your child's brain so that it becomes further integrated and the narrative can be elevated into something more meaningful and significant. Along the way you'll be teaching them to do the same so that storytelling can be a useful tool they use when they need or want it.

More and more over the coming years, your child will be out in the world, doing things independently, responding to situations based on what kind of person they are, which values they've been raised with, and how those principles influence how they think and behave. They'll face messy situations, misunderstandings, and hurt feelings. And if while you're spending regular time with them during these formative years, you focus on the stories they're telling about what they're thinking and feeling, you can narrate to integrate by guiding them to consider experiences afterward, figuring out pertinent facts and working on a repair or a resolution that sets things right.

Set Playtime Parameters

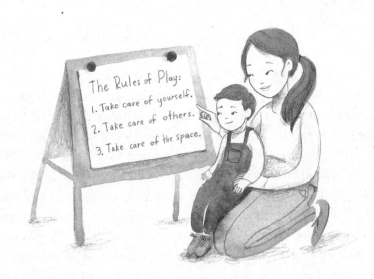

Primary skill being developed in the child:
Flexibility and adaptability to help them work within boundaries
and make positive decisions.

Primary message received by the child:
Someone is going to keep me safe and help me learn to
do that for myself.

When it comes to child-led play, parents often worry that things will get out of hand. This is a valid concern. Especially when fully engrossed in self-chosen activities, kids are going to run up against (and sometimes right through) some limits from time to time.

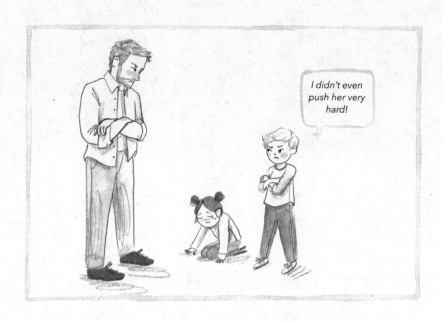

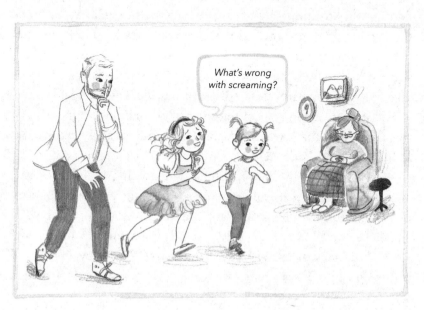

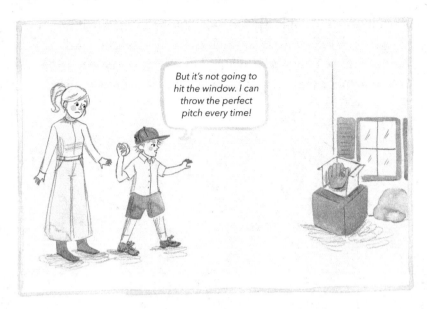

Challenges like these are one more reason play is so valuable in children's development. Virtually every single type of play involves kids learning the boundaries of what's safe and acceptable in a particular setting, figuring out how to negotiate rules everyone can agree on, learning that people won't always go along with their plan, and finding ways to cooperate toward shared goals. As Garry Landreth, the creator of child-centered play therapy, puts it, "Limits are not needed until they are needed." So when we set appropriate and well-defined boundaries that clearly communicate our expectations, we give our kids opportunities to discover new flexibility and adaptable skills they can use to respect the rules of a situation and make positive decisions. That's why a crucial PlayStrong strategy emphasizes *setting playtime parameters*.

We get it, though: Setting limits and holding boundaries isn't always fun. We hear it from parents all the time. Discipline and redirecting unwanted behaviors are consistently some of the biggest challenges we all face. Especially at the end of a long day or stressful week, kids may need and crave more freedom, movement, and expression of their emotions, and while play offers an outlet for these needs, it can also create an environment where behavior can begin to get out of hand.

Virtually every single type of play involves kids learning the boundaries of what's safe and acceptable in a particular setting, figuring out how to negotiate rules everyone can agree on, learning that people won't always go along with their plan, and finding ways to cooperate toward shared goals.

So that brings us to some questions about play:

- How can we provide our kids the kinds of play that combat stress and build stronger social emotional learning—along with all the benefits we've been describing—if we're constantly worrying that behavior will get out of control?
- What if kids get so wrapped up in the fun that they disregard basic family expectations about respecting others, taking care of toys, cleaning up afterward, and so on?
- What should we do in the moment when our child is about to cross a limit, possibly even hurting themself or someone else?

These are the types of questions we want to address here as we discuss the strategy of setting playtime parameters.

The Gift of Boundaries and Limits

It's not easy to set limits gracefully and effectively when your child is perilously poised to ride a skateboard down the staircase, or when they're aiming a soft dart gun dangerously close to your face, or when a volcano filled with red baking soda is about to explode all over the kitchen. Parents typically land somewhere between two extremes when it comes to how we'll likely handle these situations. One extreme involves being too domineering in an effort to avoid misbehavior (making up too many rules, overdirecting, shutting down child-led exploration). The other extreme is taking an overly permissive approach (being too wishy-washy about rules, not intervening enough, allowing kids to take charge even if it creates unhealthy chaos and stress).

Do you usually lean toward one of these extremes? Your answer probably depends on several dynamics, including how you were brought up, your beliefs about child development, specific cultural values about child-rearing, wider societal expectations and trends, and how you're managing to juggle family priorities. Other significant factors result from personal preferences, such as your comfort level with getting on the floor and tolerating extra sensory input like noise and messy materials.

Whether you generally believe in more or less direction and supervision of a child's play, you can still prioritize quality time playing together within healthy limits and boundaries. That way, your child can practice making respectful choices and putting on the brakes when necessary, and they can develop a robust sense of self-control and respect for others within stable, secure, and predictable relationships.

What it really comes down to is that *kids need both limits and connection,* both structure and nurturing. For the children's good, their caregivers need to set playtime parameters.

It goes without saying that your children will often react emotionally when you present a limit, whether their response is more top down (where they deliberately test the boundaries) or bottom up (where they get intensely upset, unable to think through their responses to a situation). We know that the limit-setting moment can feel stressful and unpleasant for children and parents alike, but when you work from and communicate a clearly thought-out rationale and effective formulation for when and how limit setting should occur, it can translate into powerful emotional learning for your kids.

K ids need both limits and connection, both structure and nurture.

Limits can (somewhat counterintuitively) strengthen the parent-child bond, especially once your child knows without a doubt that you're doing what's best for them, even if they don't like it. Setting limits also creates feelings of safety and predictability for the child, since they have a clear sense of how their world works—what's allowed and what's not. When you set a personal boundary, it models for them that they can set boundaries for themself with others. Plus, when you set limits, you give your kid practice putting on the brakes when they're headed in a (literal or figurative) direction that can cause trouble. This is a skill they'll need for the rest of their life. All of these benefits lead to one significant conclusion: Kids who are facing reasonable limits are kids who are learning to handle themselves well, set their own boundaries, and respect other people's boundaries.

You can see, then, why we talk about the gift of limits. *Of course* you want to prioritize your relationship with your kids. That really is what parenting is all about. But as you do so, set parameters that help them learn where the boundaries lie so they can comprehend the rules and feel safe.

The research is really clear that a domineering, command-and-demand approach to discipline doesn't provide enough connection; likewise, an overly permissive approach doesn't account for the importance of limit setting. But if we can provide *both* clear boundaries and unconditional love and connection—both structure and nurture—that's when kids can really thrive. So that's the sweet spot we want to aim for when we see unwanted behaviors during play.

> If we can provide *both* clear boundaries
> and unconditional love and connection—
> both structure and nurture—that's when
> kids can really thrive.

Before we discuss specific guidelines and strategies for confidently and lovingly setting boundaries during play, let's consider what causes kids to test their limits and engage in power struggles in the first place.

Are They Testing Limits on Purpose?

Sometimes, yes, they are—but nowhere near as often as people think. Sometimes we set limits and our kids handle it just fine. They adapt easily and realign their emotions and behaviors just as we'd hope. Then, in other moments, the most loving limit or benign boundary can send them into emotional chaos and behavioral disarray. What gives? Why the disparity—in the same kid!—between a reasonable, conscientious response in one moment and an out-of-control reaction in another?

Well, let's start there, with managing parental expectations. Testing limits is simply part of development. It's what kids do. They're *supposed* to differentiate, become individuals, find their own autonomy, explore what they're capable of, and learn how others react when they push boundaries. The development of these drives is a healthy part of a child's maturation that allows them to eventually become their own unique individual.

But the journey there isn't always a peaceful one. Because their brains are still developing, and the regulatory parts of their nervous systems are still learning their jobs, kids may react strongly at times. Sometimes those reactions will make no sense whatsoever to us.

Tina has a friend whose daughter sobbed when her mom wouldn't let her eat the Band-Aid on her scraped knee. For a good laugh, and to feel some parental validation, perform an internet search for the multitude of stories parents tell about the kinds of things their kids have melted down about. (*But why can't I climb down the chimney like Santa?!*)

If you're expecting consistent rationality and comprehensible behavior from your children, or you expect that they'll unswervingly work *within* the boundaries instead of *against* them, then your starting place is a developmentally inappropriate expectation (especially for little kids). Instead, assume they will test and cross boundaries, and know that when they do, it's a healthy part of development. Do you need to address it even though it's part of childhood? Definitely! But if you expect perfect behavior all the time, you're asking for disappointment.

What's more, what appears as disobedience to us isn't usually meant to be a deliberate misbehavior by a child. They aren't always thinking in a logical, top-down way about the consequences of their actions in a state of play. Too many times we mistake a child's well-intended, purely natural, creative impulses as intentional misconduct simply because what they do catches us off guard or doesn't fit our preconceived notions of how kids *should* behave.

> Too many times we mistake a child's well-intended, purely natural, creative impulses as intentional misconduct simply because what they do catches us off guard or doesn't fit our preconceived notions of how kids *should* behave.

A mess to a parent might be a work of art to a child. Likewise, children's impulses might appear to us as disorganized, immature, or uncontrollable, but those actions are often completely necessary, normal, creative, and healthy. These are the very moments that are architecting your child's brain and providing ample opportunities for development to proceed in an individually determined, yet predictable, set of stages. When our kids are young, they are biologically programmed to experiment, test their abilities, and push the limits of what they *can* do. It just takes a lot longer to develop good judgment about whether they *should or shouldn't* do it.

A MESS TO A PARENT MIGHT BE A WORK OF ART TO A CHILD.

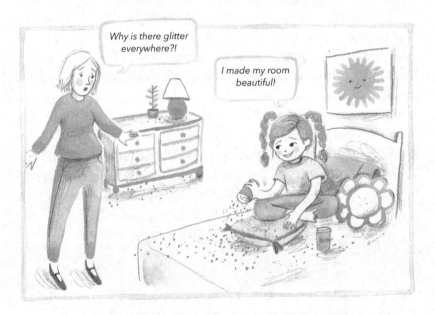

Even as kids get older, you'll see them push back against limits: when they're facing tough challenges, not feeling their best, storing up lots of emotional tension, dealing with sensory and developmental differences, or running a bit too hot in their intensity thermostat and losing their grip on calm regulation.

This isn't necessarily a bad thing. Not at all. One of the biggest advantages of child-led unstructured play is that it provides a creative outlet to release pent-up energy and emotional overflow so that it doesn't erupt in undesirable behavior at the wrong times or when the demands or consequences are higher. So think of your child's open-ended play with you as a "safe container": a supportive, even therapeutic, space where we can find some value in a child's desire to break a limit, then use these moments to help them learn to manage their frustrations and other difficult emotions more effectively.

> Think of your child's open-ended play with you as a "safe container": a supportive, even therapeutic, space where we can find some value in a child's desire to break a limit, then use these moments to help them learn to manage their frustrations and other difficult emotions more effectively.

Ideally, when you create those feelings of safety for your kids, they'll know they can push back against boundaries without risking losing your love. Assuming that's where things stand in the parent-child relationship, there are lots of reasons kids test limits. Sometimes they're genuinely unclear on what the rules are. Or maybe they know the rules but are just working from a still-developing prefrontal cortex that may not be thoroughly considering the ramifications and consequences of their actions, either for themselves or for someone else. At times, especially for younger children, they might simply be curious about the effects of certain actions rather than intentionally deciding to misbehave.

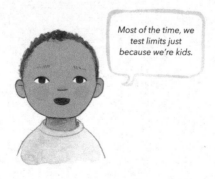

Most of the time, we test limits just because we're kids.

To go even further, it's really important to know that what may seem like an intentional misbehavior can actually be a child experiencing an overwhelming stress response, where they have simply become emotionally dysregulated. In other words, sometimes they actually *can't* "use their words" or "make a good choice." They need your help to move back into a calmer and more composed state. And again, most of these reasons are completely developmentally healthy.

I NEED CLARITY ON THE RULES.

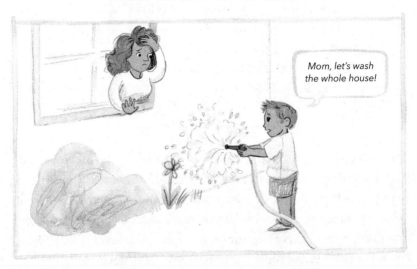

I'M CURIOUS ABOUT WHAT MIGHT HAPPEN.

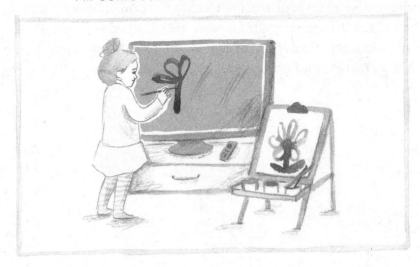

I NEED YOU TO HELP ME GET CALM AGAIN.

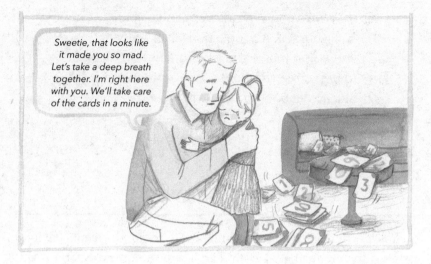

When you really think about it, the vast majority of the time that kids test limits, they're doing it for a reason other than to willfully misbehave. Instead, they're unclear and unaware of the consequences, or they're curious, or they're simply upset beyond their ability to control their feelings and actions. Sometimes kids do make intentional decisions to break a rule, but that happens far less often than most parents think. And even when it does happen, the kid often has a pretty good reason why they made that decision. If you'll spend a few minutes connecting with them first, then the rest of the discipline process (which, again, is all about teaching, not punishment) will go much more smoothly.

None of this means that you don't still maintain your boundaries. Doing so may be even *more* important in these situations. But first, *chase the why* and remain curious yourself. Ask questions like, "Why is she doing that?" You'll be much more likely to get to the root of the issue and then be able to respond more lovingly *and effectively*.

Chase the why and remain curious yourself. Ask questions like, "Why is she doing that?" You'll be much more likely to get to the root of the issue and then be able to respond more lovingly *and effectively.*

The Rules of Play

So how do you figure out when and how to respond when behavioral issues come up during play? And are there certain expectations you want to prioritize over others?

Yes, there are. We call them the rules of play.

You can share these guidelines with your kids, and they're pretty good principles for wherever and however they're playing: by themselves, with you and/or siblings, on playdates or at recess, and so on. The rules are simple enough that they'll make sense to children of any age, and they're based on the message play therapists usually give their young clients when they first start working together: "We don't hurt ourselves or others, we try not to break the toys or space on purpose (although accidents might happen), and if there's anything else you're not allowed to do, I'll let you know." Clearly articulated boundaries like these are what the rules of play offer.

Rule #1: Take care of yourself

Children want to feel that we trust them to make good choices as they play, but sometimes they'll need us to help them stay safe. When we refer to taking care of yourself, this is primarily about safety. Some kids (depending on their age, developmental level, or specific individual differences) may need more scaffolding and support in this area. Limit setting comes into play when an activity creates too much risk of injury to a child's body or emotional sense of safety.

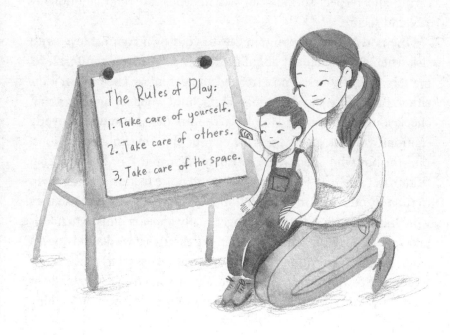

You'd likely step in, in other words, if your kid is about to hit himself on the head with a toy, bump into a mirror, jump off a high set of stairs, or follow the next YouTube link into who-knows-what cyberspace. Same for playing with sharp or breakable objects, applying paint near her eyes or mouth, or inspecting the electrical outlet with tweezers. Kids may not like it when you enforce a boundary, but they do feel more *secure* when you set some limitations on their behavior.

Doing so also protects them from feeling excessive shame or guilt about hurting others when we intervene before someone gets injured. Stopping a child from throwing objects at a friend during a playdate prevents not only bumps and bruises but also the worry, embarrassment, or rejection they might feel after hurting someone. We can't always prevent children from hitting or throwing things when they're angry, but as a rule, setting limits can be an act of genuine parental caring and respect so kids can remain physically and emotionally safe and secure.

One note: Avoid stepping in due to your own comfort level with risk when it's not actually about the child's safety. Your comfort level matters, too, of course, and a freaked-out parent isn't helpful for kids, either. But before you jump in and set a limit when it's not necessary, check yourself. If you tend to run on the anxious side and to be overly cautious, you risk losing the trust of your child in similar situations. Like the boy who cried wolf, our call to "Be careful" or to warn them "That's not safe" can become background noise to kids, leading them to tune us out. And that, in fact, makes them *less* safe because they won't take us seriously when danger really appears. Plus, when kids take safe-enough risks, it allows them to learn what works and doesn't work, and it allows them to be wiser and even safer in the years to come. So when you get worried about something your child is doing, ask yourself, "Is this really unsafe, or is my own anxiety taking over?"

Rule #2: Take care of others

We've discussed empathy at several points throughout the book, and here is one more time that play offers the opportunity to teach kids to consider the feelings of the people around them. When we talk about taking care of others, we don't mean to teach children that they are somehow *responsible* for how other people feel or experience the world; that message leads to codependence and unhealthy relationships. We're just choosing simple language to let kids know that they want to consider how their actions can impact the people they interact with.

It's important that they learn that certain behaviors aren't acceptable, including ones that threaten to hurt someone else, either physically or emotionally. You might tell your child, for example, that it's not OK to flick paint at someone's face, or call a sibling mean names, or use a toy to hit someone. You may have to make it clear that there are rules against using the family dog as a horse. These are limits that continue to teach and communicate about choices, consequences, and empathy.

Rule #3: Take care of the space

Part of the emotional security we offer children when we play involves giving them a set of consistent expectations about what's safe and acceptable in the space or environment we occupy. Consistency is uniquely important to the process of learning to care for the rooms and outdoor places we play in, as well as the toys and materials in them. Accidents are bound to happen, but smashing and breaking toys on purpose wouldn't be acceptable. Wasting materials, like pouring out an entire bottle of glue, can be costly. Destroying or damaging floors, walls, or furniture should be prevented, but making some messes that can be cleaned up together or fixing objects broken by accident is absolutely part of healthy play.

Most of these examples may seem obvious, but because we frequently get questions from parents about how permissive they should be in a free, unstructured play environment, we want to be specific about how much freedom is really allowed. Whether you're observing top-down activity (which is under your child's conscious control) or more dysregulated bottom-up (and therefore unintentional) behavior, you want to prevent damage to the physical space and protect the playthings in it so that the toys and materials can remain available and stay in good shape as long as possible.

In this way, children once again experience the security of knowing that we'll be consistent. They learn how to take care of belongings, and they develop deeper respect and responsibility for their surrounding environment and the home you share as a family— a respect that can then be applied in settings outside your home.

One warning: Don't let the rules become the point. These are guidelines meant to help you set clear boundaries, but you don't want them to dominate the parent-child relationship and affect the overall benefits your child is getting from playing with you. In other words, the rules of play create a developmentally sound set of expectations, or structure, for your playtimes and map out where the boundaries are for your child ahead of time.

> **D**on't let the rules become the point.
> These are guidelines meant to help you
> set clear boundaries, but you don't want
> them to dominate the parent-child
> relationship and affect the overall benefits
> your child is getting from playing with you.

But they aren't priorities to focus on constantly, and we don't advise making up a long list of dos and don'ts, or watching like a hawk in case kids do something wrong. You don't want to limit so much of your child's creative spark that it ceases to even feel like play. The rules are simple, straightforward statements that offer healthy parent-child connection and reinforce our number one job as parents—to keep our children safe—and provide the necessary structure to build our kids' decision-making skills within the creative space that play provides.

Be the Pit Crew, Not the Race Engineer

Just as we don't want to make the rules the whole point, it's important not to take over when we play with our kids. Instead, we want to let them lead.

Play follows the law of inertia. A child's body in motion wants to remain in motion. To varying degrees, we do need to interrupt, intervene, or redirect when we see a problem, but instead of shutting the whole thing down, we recommend merging into the flow of the play and supporting where it needs to go. If play is becoming unsafe, or your child is too dysregulated, then by all means pause the action immediately so you can help.

But if you're about to say no, or some version of it, take a second before you say it. *Stop yelling. Don't run with scissors. No playing ball in the house. You're going to spill.* We often deliver these commands automatically, without thinking about their effects. But the truth is, using the word "no" may lead your child to push back against your limit with even more force. In our experience, top-down limit-setting phrases—like "no," "don't," "you can't," "stop that," "you're not allowed to"—often press the gas pedal on kids' desire to prove they were right to do what they did, or it causes them to wait and do it again later when your back is turned. Even as adults, we may have the impulse to push back when someone tells us we can't do something!

Instead, look to position yourself differently to keep your child in the flow of playful learning. Rather than issuing commands from the sidelines like a Formula 1 race engineer, come in like a member of a pit crew. The race engineer dictates everything the race car should (and shouldn't) do, whereas the pit crew's strategy is different. They take a team approach, pumping up the driver or offering more fuel to get back on track within seconds. A pit-crew parent doesn't need to spend a lot of time explaining, lecturing, and telling kids exactly what to do—their goal is to barely cause a ripple in the flow of learning.

That's not always easy when it comes to parenting, though. When children argue, stonewall, talk back, and refuse to do what we ask, it often leads to a challenging pattern of mental rigidity that's hard for everyone to break out of, kids and parents alike. Ever notice that the more rigid your child becomes, the more rigid you often get? And vice versa? Instead, dismantle those walls and build up the relationship so you can elicit kids' cooperation by affirming their play—their most intrinsic, motivational, developmental drive.

Pit-crew parents notice when their child is stuck in a behavior. They draw physically near and crouch or bend to the child's level (if not lower), and they offer encouragement to set things in a positive direction. What stimulates cooperation and creativity in this moment? Connection. It's the fuel for playful learning.

When your child runs into a limit, it helps enormously if you come across as more of a teammate than a competitor or adversary. That means your child feels a certain satisfaction when you hop into the pit with them to deal with the issue. It's harder to accomplish when you've had to put the brakes on a challenging behavior and your child is angry with you, but it's still possible in that situation—and very helpful—to position yourself as an ally. It's a powerful statement when you lean over and whisper, "Hey, buddy, I'm on your side. Let's look at this together. Where do we go from here? We've got this."

FIRST: INSTEAD OF SETTING LIMITS LIKE A RACE ENGINEER . . .

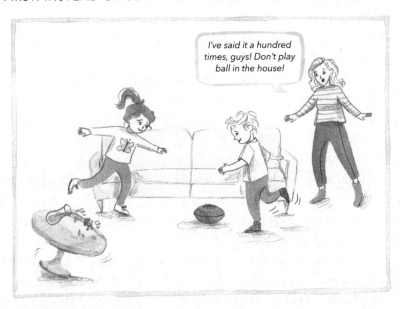

SECOND: SET LIMITS LIKE A PIT CREW.

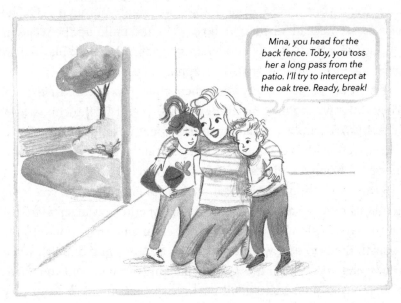

Set Playtime Parameters: Step by Step

Once you've set the right tone, aiming always for connection, you can move in and address the unwanted behavior. This strategy is similar to the approach set down years ago by Garry Landreth, and it can allow you to set limits with more ease while conveying care and acceptance for your child's desires, needs, and feelings.

Step 1: Observe and attune

As always, your first step is to really see your child and chase the why. Allow that perception to help you understand what's going on within them, below the surface—what's really driving them to act in this way? Having a better understanding of where your child is, both emotionally and in terms of their desires, can make the entire discipline process much more smooth.

Step 2: Acknowledge the desire

Next, communicate what you've noticed. Let your child know that you're attuned to them by delivering a message that says "You are seen." Communicate that you understand the feeling, desire, need, or motive—in short, *the why*—behind the behavior.

You might say something like, "I can tell how mad you are that she didn't give you your turn to try to score a goal" or "You really want to spray your sister" or "That was really disappointing, wasn't it, that we had to stop playing just now." Starting off with the message "you are seen" sets the stage for safety so kids can learn more acceptable ways of communicating feelings.

When children feel seen and understood, the reason for the behavior can often come into focus and help mitigate the need for further limit setting. When it comes to anger, especially, simply acknowledging the feeling with empathy can dial down the intensity and reduce destructiveness. Kids will often drop what they were about to do, such as throwing a toy, because a caring adult has named and accepted their emotions.

This might remind you of an earlier strategy in the book—Think Out Loud, which is very similar to what you're doing in this step.

Speaking first to your child's deeper thoughts, feelings, needs, and intentions provides a basis for developing a wider emotional vocabulary and builds emotional intelligence, creating a safe environment for play to adapt to limits and structure.

Step 3: Set the limit

Once you've connected with your child and let them know that you're clear on what they're experiencing and feeling, then explain the limit that you're setting. Doing so might mean saying, "It's OK to feel mad, but it's not OK to hit or hurt others" or "I can see how frustrated that makes you, but we want to have time to read, so it's time to brush your teeth now."

Without activating shame, you want to explain the limit in as few words as possible, using language that offers empathy. Limits should be specific and totally clear about what's acceptable or allowed and what's not.

And as often as possible, be playful *while* you're setting limits. Being silly or lighthearted is a great way to gain cooperation and impose boundaries. It can make battles—like buckling seatbelts, completing homework, shutting off devices, and so on—much more manageable. It can help us as parents respond to difficult moments with less reactivity while also building fun memories, shared moments, and inside jokes. It's so much more fun than a battle over toothbrushing to pull out some silliness: "What's that, Mr. Plaque? You want to stay in Emily's mouth so you can try to make a cavity? Don't worry, you *might* be able to stay in there, because I don't see her toothbrush in her hand." Or if your kid is into nature, pretend the toothbrush is a submarine, searching for deep sea monsters, and then ham it up a little bit: "Oh my goodness, I think your tooth-sub just found the formidable seapizzafish!"

Or set a timer for ten minutes of homework, then tell your child to come sneak up on you and see if they can scare you after the timer goes off.

One time Tina's son was feeling overwhelmed by five notecards he had to fill out for homework. She told him to bring her each notecard after it was done (getting him to get up and move his body) and that she would do something to try to make him laugh after each card. He was determined not to laugh, but eventually she got him giggling because she was trying so hard.

Simply by using silly voices, pretending, or getting into a playful state ourselves, we can often help our kids follow rules and expectations without exhausting ourselves or having to engage in major battles.

Step 4: Offer alternatives

Kids are firing on all cylinders when they play—mentally and emotionally—so it can be really hard for them to immediately stop what they're doing and shift gears. At this step of limit setting, parents should follow the law of inertia and realize that it's much easier to direct your child into a lane of acceptable behavior than to bring them to a sudden, gear-grinding stop.

What better way to build the skills of self-control than giving some power back to your child? That's what you'll be doing when you ask, "Where could you build Legos that the baby can't reach them?" Depending on where kids are in their development and abilities, they may need a pair of alternatives presented to them because they aren't yet able to come up with different options on the spot: "Would you rather build Legos on the table or the kitchen counter?" Either way, you get the Legos off the floor while still allowing your child some agency, even if they're upset about having to move their emerging creation.

Combine this final step with the others, and a limit-setting moment can go much more smoothly. For example, imagine that you hear a distant shriek from the room where your two sons are playing. You hurry there and see your six-year-old standing in the doorway, blocking the way out for his younger brother, who is holding a dinosaur possessively in his arms. You know what you *don't* want the boys to do—fight over the dinosaur. But how do you help resolve the situation? How do you guide your older son into a lane of acceptable behavior and empower him to make good decisions?

First, you observe and attune—and you'd better be quick, because things are rapidly escalating. Luckily, it doesn't take more than a second to see that your younger son, Peter, has once again claimed one of his brother's toys for himself, and his big brother is about to explode.

STEP 1: OBSERVE AND ATTUNE.

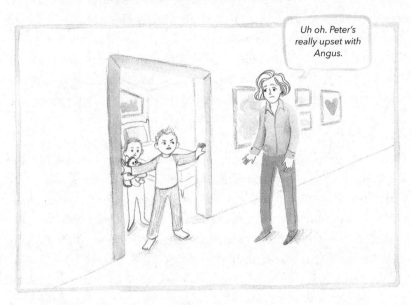

Having noticed the state that Peter's in, it's time to get his attention and try to move toward resolving the conflict by empathetically acknowledging and naming his emotions, motives, and desires.

STEP 2: ACKNOWLEDGE THE DESIRE.

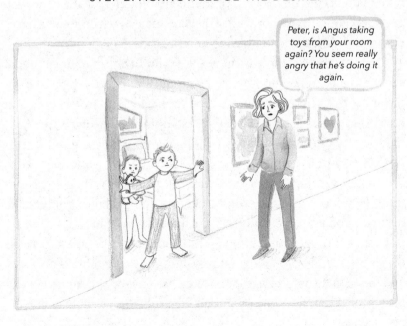

Now it's time to set the limit, doing so as clearly as possible and using as few words as you can.

STEP 3: SET THE LIMIT.

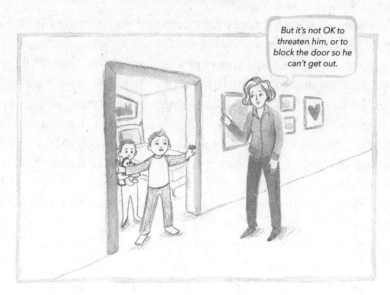

Then offer an alternative. Look for a way to invite Peter's thinking brain into the moment so that he can make a better choice.

STEP 4: OFFER ALTERNATIVES.

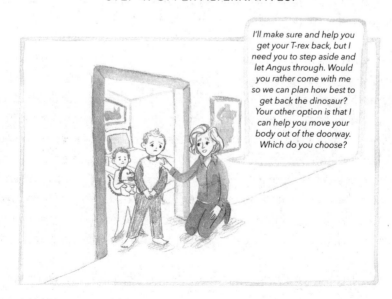

Notice that in this scenario, the mom offers Peter loving empathy, and she still set a clear expectation. She's ultimately the authority figure here, and that's important. But she does all she can to express herself with care and respect.

Observe, too, that she worked straight through the steps in order. That won't always happen. You may not be able to follow this sequence every time. Doing so isn't always practically possible. Some children express a heightened sensitivity when they're feeling dysregulated in their bodies, and reflecting their feelings back to them only makes things worse. *Don't tell me how I feel! You don't know!* Reflecting their feelings is the opposite of what some kids need when they're upset. Instead of creating more safety, it seems to exacerbate their stress responses and cause more aggression. So you might choose to skip the step of validating their emotions. If you're connecting with them about how you imagine that they feel, it's helpful to use language that lets them know that you're aware that you might not be exactly right about their experience. Try using words and phrases like "It seems like . . ." and "You look [name the emotion]. Is that right?" As always, do your best to avoid one-size-fits-all approaches, and instead, attune to this one child in this one moment.

There will also be times when the urgency of the situation—your child is about to hurt themself or someone else, or break something, for example—may require us to skip straight to the limit setting. Prioritize creating safe conditions and supporting your child through co-regulation, where stating the limit can help to explain why you need to provide more containment.

For example, if your child is angrily trying to smash her dollhouse, it would be very reasonable for you to gently, but firmly, block her access to the toy and say, "I'm going to be right here to keep both you and the dollhouse safe." When she has returned to a calmer state, that would be a better time to validate how she may have been feeling and to help her reflect on the experience: "It looked like you were so mad that the dolls kept falling over. That's why you were angry with the dollhouse? I can see that you're feeling calmer now. What should we try next?"

Don't think you have to robotically or formulaically work your way through the steps every time your child needs help regulating themself. Just get clear on what the steps are, then let common sense and your love for your child guide you.

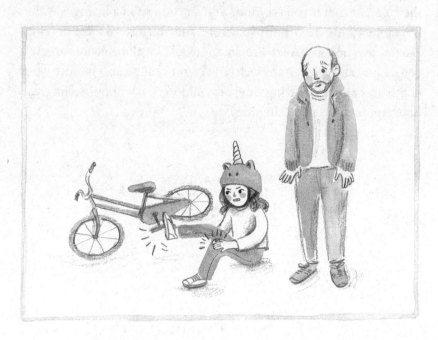

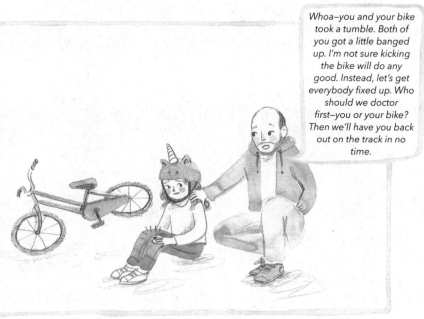

Always keep in mind: You can be warm and empathetic even as you set limits, saying yes to your child even as you say no to a behavior. Sometimes people think that if you're warm you can't also enforce the rules, or that if you set limits you can't do so in a loving way. But remember, kids need both structure and nurture. As the developmental psychologist Aliza Pressman says, "Not all behaviors are welcome, but all feelings are welcome." You really can embrace your child, and all their feelings, desires, and needs, without feeling you must approve of everything they do.

YOU CAN BE WARM AND EMPATHETIC
EVEN AS YOU SET LIMITS, SAYING YES TO YOUR CHILD
EVEN AS YOU SAY NO TO A BEHAVIOR.

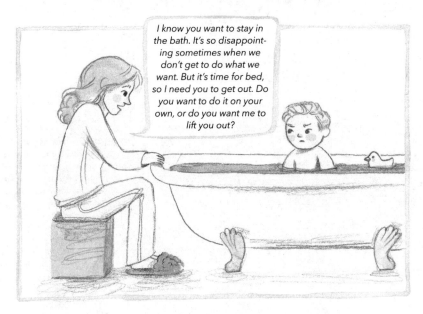

Dealing with Tantrums

Setting playtime parameters should be about helping kids go *through* emotions, not around them. If you discover that after presenting a limit, your child has a big reactive meltdown because you're not allowing a behavior, focus on being the safe container they need. That means helping and supporting them as they move back into regulation, and first addressing their emotional needs (or their hunger, fatigue, sensory overload, or any other reason they might be melting down). Sitting with them quietly, offering your lap, breathing deeply, and other forms of calm connection should be your first line of defense when kids are too dysregulated to playfully reengage.

When your child calms down to the point that they're sniffling instead of screaming, that's when playful redirection can come in really handy: "Would you like to blow some bubbles? Find all the blue things in this room? Pick flowers and make a bouquet?" That kind of redirection can help a child shift into a more receptive state where they can absorb new skills and add self-regulatory tools to their tool kit.

Setting Limits: When It's Time to Stop Playing

Transitions can be tough for kids, and one of the hardest is when it's time for play to stop. Transitioning from playing and moving into doing something else involves limit setting around time. When you support them with this type of transition, you're actually assisting your child as they learn the valuable life skills of planning ahead, managing time, and delaying gratification. Kids have to figure out how to bring an activity to a stopping point, leave a task unfinished, finish what they can, manage anxiety, let go of enjoyment, and hold on to ideas until the next play session. That's a lot to ask of a kid, but these are all major milestones in cognitive development that take years to master. It's developmentally normal for kids to stall, whine, act like they didn't hear you, or even (*Wait, one more thing!*) beg for more time.

Kids have to figure out how to bring an activity to a stopping point, leave a task unfinished, finish what they can, manage anxiety, let go of enjoyment, and hold on to ideas until the next play session. That's a lot to ask of a kid, but these are all major milestones in cognitive development that take years to master. It's developmentally normal for kids to stall, whine, act like they didn't hear you, or even (*Wait, one more thing!*) beg for more time.

It's really important to acknowledge the monumental skill building that's happening while kids take a few extra minutes to transition successfully. Here are a few transition tips for parents trying to help kids stop the play.

Transition tip #1: It's not supposed to be smooth and seamless
Transitions are usually bumpy at first. It takes a while to learn a new routine, but with some repetition, kids do get on board. Remember the law of inertia? Kids don't come equipped to make quick stops when they're playing. So allow a few minutes—and give your child a warning—to create a "stopping place" that they can see coming.

Transition tip #2: Don't just set a timer; create an ending ritual
Yes, talk to your child at the five-minute warning. But also ask them how they'd prefer to bring their activity to a close. What would they like to do in their final five minutes? Which loose ends need to be tied up? Can they think of this part as one chapter in a longer story? Perhaps a younger child wants to tuck her stuffed animals into bed, or an older child wants to take a bow and receive applause as the curtain closes on his musical performance. Let kids practice getting closure each time they play.

Transition tip #3: Accept disappointment

Despite all your best efforts, and even if you've memorized every word of this book, kids are still going to act in ways you wish they wouldn't. Play transports children to imaginary worlds where they lose track of time and reality. Kids often remark to Georgie at the end of a play therapy session, "It's over already?" They might be hot, sweaty, tired, and ready for a break after playing a game of tag for a solid hour—but suggest stopping and you'll hear a resounding "No!"

You know how kids start complaining toward the end of a fun day out? Are they actually mad they didn't get that hot dog–shaped balloon they wanted, or is it more likely they had a blast playing and they're already missing being there? It can help to acknowledge their disappointment and reassure them it's normal to feel that way when enjoyable things end. It also feels good to appreciate experiences and start looking forward to the next fun activity.

But still, all that said, we're setting ourselves up for a lot of frustration if we expect kids not to become upset when it's time to end an activity they're thoroughly enjoying. Keep in mind that it's OK if your kids feel angry or disappointed or sad. Especially with regulated parents who allow them to feel while holding boundaries, kids can practice working through their emotions, thus building their capacity to work through big feelings and adversity in the future. One of Tina's frequent phrases with her boys was "It's hard to feel disappointed. I'm right here with you while you're feeling it." We don't have to give in or change the boundary. We allow them to feel, and we offer connection, even during these upset moments.

Transition tip #4: Plan a transitional activity that's almost as much fun

Some children just can't make an easy shift from a highly preferred activity to one that requires more sustained attention. There's a big difference between bouncing on a trampoline and sitting down to concentrate on double-digit multiplication homework. We've found that inserting a brief transitional activity helps kids make the switch between preferred and nonpreferred activities, like spending a few minutes playing a card game, drawing a picture, telling jokes, dancing around the kitchen, or making a snack together. The trick is to find an in-between, "just right" activity that assists your child to make the mental shift into more dedicated attention and focus, like playing a math *game* as a warm-up for harder problems.

TRANSITIONAL ACTIVITIES CAN HELP
WHEN IT'S TIME TO STOP PLAYING.

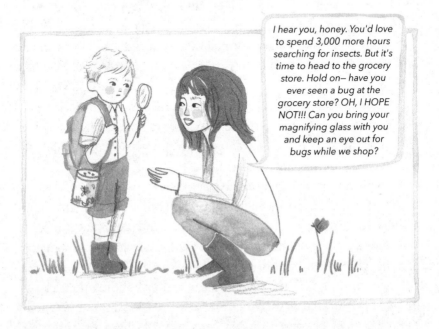

Transition tip #5: Set limits with confident momentum

When play must be paused to take care of other pressing priorities, the limit-setting techniques we've outlined here should be helpful. Feeling comfortable being the grown-up in charge, and being consistent with limits, allows children to trust us so they can move forward more effectively.

In the end, we parents have to accept that dysregulation is going to come with play. It just is. And that means you're going to have to set playtime parameters. That's the bad news. But the good news is that play is so often *also* the antidote to upset feelings. It can completely change the mood of a child and the overall emotional tone of a parent-child interaction. So when you play with your child, don't be surprised when some negative interactions crop up from time to time. When they do, just work through the steps outlined above—observe and attune, acknowledge the desire, set the limit, and offer alternatives—and you'll be on your way to moving back toward regulation and teaching your child invaluable skills along the way.

Be Playful Beyond
the Playroom

Our primary focus throughout *The Way of Play* has been on how you can help your kids grow and develop by spending a few minutes each day playing with them. We started with the Think Out Loud strategy, where you simply name what you see your child doing, thus taking the first steps toward showing them that it's possible to pay attention to another person's mind—which means they can pay attention to their own thoughts and intentions as well. Then we moved to Make Yourself a Mirror, where you reflect back the actions of your child so they can feel you tuning in to them and paying attention to their emotional life, and then they learn to do the same with people around them. The next PlayStrong strategy, Bring Emotions to Life, builds on the first two, focusing explicitly on helping kids recognize, manage, and express their feelings.

Kids will often need help in that process, so the fourth strategy, Dial Intensity Up or Down, focuses on "chasing the why" when you notice outsized (or undersized) responses to difficult situations and then looking for ways to bring calmness or energy to a situation. The next PlayStrong strategy, Scaffold and Stretch, gets specific about skills you can build in your kids by providing the support (scaffolding) they need, while challenging (stretching) them to deal with more difficult moments. Another way to help your kids handle fears, deal with conflict, and understand themselves is to use storytime to Narrate to Integrate, our sixth PlayStrong strategy. And finally, Set Playtime Parameters, the strategy you just read about, stresses the importance of establishing appropriate and well-defined boundaries that clearly communicate your expectations while prioritizing, pretty much above all else, the loving relationship you share with your kids.

Now, as we close, we want to make the overarching point that the power of play can extend far beyond the playroom. You can use play and playfulness in an almost limitless number of ways as you interact with and relate to your children. Play can elevate experiences shared with your kids and teach them skills to make life much, much easier, especially when it comes to gaining their cooperation for less enjoyable daily tasks and routines.

By inserting more playful solutions into challenging everyday situations with your kids—to elicit your child's cooperation, help them shift out of a negative mood, make a necessary chore feel more fun, and on and on—you can decrease the conflict in your relationship while also holding boundaries. This sets your child up for better motivation and self-direction when confronted with the difficult tasks of life.

> By inserting more playful solutions into challenging everyday situations with your kids ... you can decrease the conflict in your relationship while also holding boundaries. This sets your child up for better motivation and self-direction when confronted with the difficult tasks of life.

Along the way, you may find that far beyond alleviating the stress of getting our kids to join in with tasks they dislike or handling discipline moments, playfulness becomes much more a part of who we are as parents—and not simply something that we do.

The Playful Pathway

All parents can feel frustrated and powerless when a child is stalling or pushing back against structure or routine. That's especially the case when these daily tasks are not new, are fairly simple to complete, and are actually intended to provide children with good care and nurturing—like helping them get enough sleep, eat nourishing meals, do well in school, avoid too much screen time, and have some time left over to enjoy as a family. It can also lead to more dysregulated feelings, for children and parents alike, when kids are grumpy, overtired, late for school, fighting homework, and arguing about rules or basics like chores, hygiene, safety, nutrition, family responsibilities, and so on.

It may be that play is the last thing you'd even consider when conflict comes up between you and your kids. But the truth is, it can be one of your most powerful tools. We're not talking about forgetting boundaries or rules or dropping everything and throwing out parental norms and age-appropriate expectations. Sure, there may be a time to say, "Let's put your homework aside for a bit. Grab a Frisbee and we'll head to the park!"

But that's not what we're suggesting with the PlayStrong approach. We're talking about using play as an effective way to deal with conflict and connect with your child when they're stuck in a difficult moment—if they're shut down, flooded with emotion, uncooperative, or even adversarial with you—and nothing else is working. We've had parents in our offices tell us that they don't want to do a puppet show just to get their kid to put on their bleeping shoes, and we have felt that kind of exasperation ourselves. In other words, it can be cognitively exhausting to feel like you have to tap into creativity and think of being silly or inventive or playful in those moments.

And you certainly don't want to feel like you have to be *performing* for your kid all the time.

The truth, though, is that the more we bring playfulness into our daily interactions with our kids, the easier and more automatic it becomes, requiring fewer and fewer mental resources. And, summoning a bit of silliness in tough moments with your kids can be far less demanding and time-consuming than engaging in a battle of the wills. Playfulness can be just the thing to shift out of conflict, pushback, and disconnection, creating instead an environment where your child can let go of their own fears and frustrations and step into more playful connection to work *with* you.

> Playfulness can be just the thing to shift out of conflict, pushback, and disconnection, creating instead an environment where your child can let go of their own fears and frustrations and step into more playful motivation to work *with* you.

Are there times when you have to simply pick your child up off the floor, grab their shoes, and say, "It's time to leave—we need to go now"? Yes, definitely. We're not saying you need to be a playful ball of fun 24-7. That would be inauthentic and exhausting, not to mention impossible.

But the fact is that play, even in moments of great difficulty, can often make things easier on you as well as create a much stronger connection between you and your kids. If you've already developed a connected presence by playing with them on a regular basis, wouldn't it be only natural to approach parent-child challenges from the same position?

Tina had a ten-year-old client, we'll call her Emmy, who had some sensory processing challenges. Her mom's presence was her best strategy for staying regulated, so when it was time for her mom to leave, even when Emmy was with her safe, fun dad, she became so anxious her stomach would hurt, and she would have a major meltdown, which was stressful for her, her siblings, her mom, and her dad.

Emmy's nervous system created an association between her mom leaving and feelings of panic. In an effort to help Emmy change this association, Tina and Emmy prepared for an upcoming night when Emmy's mom had a PTA meeting. They planned how she and her siblings could prank and play practical jokes on their dad. Emmy and her siblings compiled a large laundry basket full of socks, put Dad's underwear in the freezer, and put a fake bug in his salad. When it was time for Mom to leave and she put her hand on the doorknob, when Emmy would typically become panicked, this time she looked forward to that moment. Mom gave Emmy the signal that meant it was time to launch Operation Prank Dad, and the great sock attack could begin. The anticipation of fun, and the playfulness and laughter of that moment (not to mention how great it was for the siblings to work together for a common goal), allowed Emmy to tolerate the anxiety and discomfort she felt with Mom leaving. It's these kinds of play states that allow our kids not only to handle themselves better in the moment but also to practice and expand their skills and resilience. And even more remarkable, when these new and positive associations get repeated, they can begin to shape the automatic associations in the brain.

Shift into a playful approach with your kids when they're having a hard time following instructions or cooperating—when you need to get them into the car, defuse a conflict between siblings, keep voices down, or have them *walk* with you instead of sprinting off. Tap into the shared language you've already cultivated, and use playfulness to help accomplish your parenting goals: not just to solve momentary problems and gain compliance but also, in the long run, to teach your child skills and give them practice balancing their desires and wishes with what's being asked of them. Instead of communicating threat or that you're on opposing sides, use play and playfulness to communicate safety, connection, and joining together.

The Playful Pivot

Imagine a moment in your own household that frequently causes discord between you and your child.

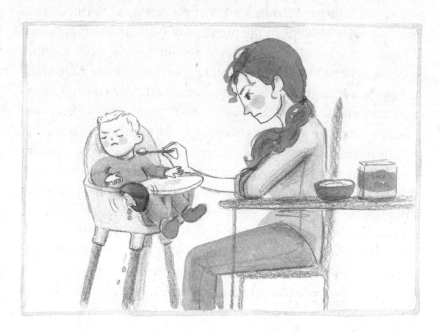

What if in this moment, instead of seeing an exasperated or even angry parent, your child received a surprisingly playful response: a gleam in your eye, a lilt in your voice, and a hint of silliness in your approach? Wouldn't approaching the situation in this manner change the entire interaction? Your kid would be expecting one response, but you'd offer something entirely different. Instead of putting up their guard or digging in their heels, they'll be more likely to relax and possibly even lean in to the task between you. That's the playful pivot.

Why pivot? Because it's usually far more effective in helping your child work with you and in keeping you both emotionally regulated. Plus, it can completely change the dynamics in the current moment and adjust what's happening inside your child's mind. After all, if their behavior seems disorganized on the outside, chances are that they're feeling a lack of control on the inside, too. Therefore, the way we understand and respond to minor hiccups can help them once again get organized and engaged—both externally and internally—when they've fallen out of sync.

Getting into a synchronous flow means finding ways to make the interaction positive. Scientists say that the feel-good hormone oxytocin is largely at work in the presence of positive emotion, as the different branches of the autonomic nervous system work together to create better synchrony. Interestingly, oxytocin is one of the hormones that's thought to stimulate parent-child closeness and bonding from birth, so it seems uniquely suited to help us achieve a better state of connection when kids of any age aren't syncing with us.

Put simply, our kids are more likely to calmly receive our attempts to address conflicts and resistance in an oxytocin-rich environment. And what stimulates more of that amazing hormone that can markedly increase your child's receptivity? Warmth, physical affection, and positive words of encouragement. And, of course, play.

That's why you initiate the playful pivot. Turning toward fun and laughter can make all the difference, whether you're trying to encourage cooperation, help with a transition, or move through and beyond conflict.

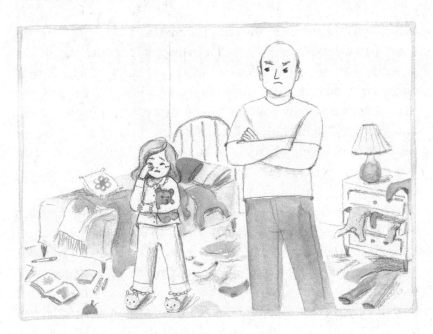

HELP YOUR CHILD PIVOT PLAYFULLY INTO COOPERATION.

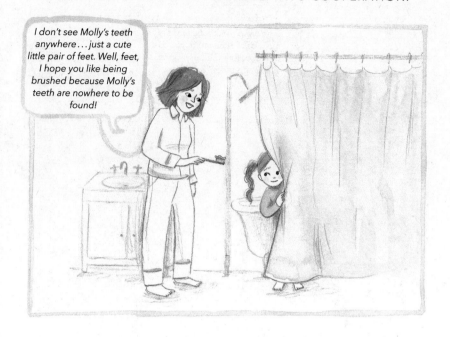

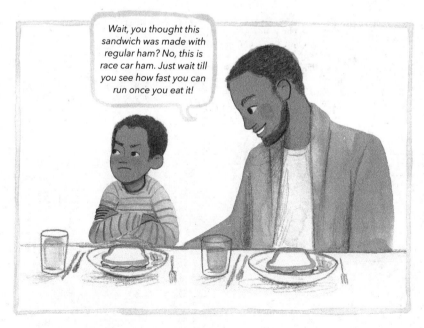

HELP YOUR CHILD PIVOT PLAYFULLY INTO A TRANSITION.

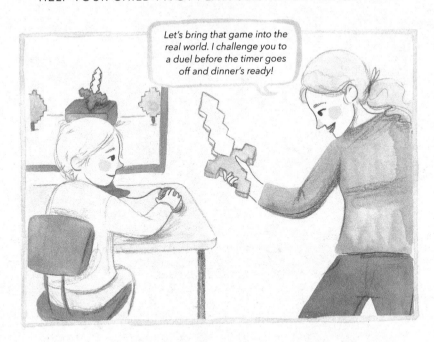

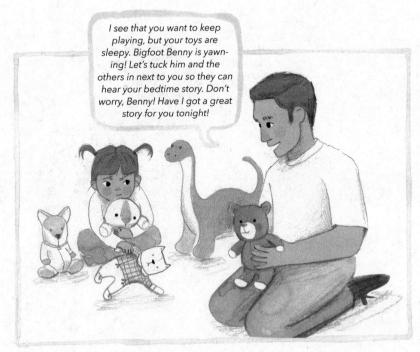

HELP YOUR CHILD PIVOT PLAYFULLY AWAY FROM CONFLICT.

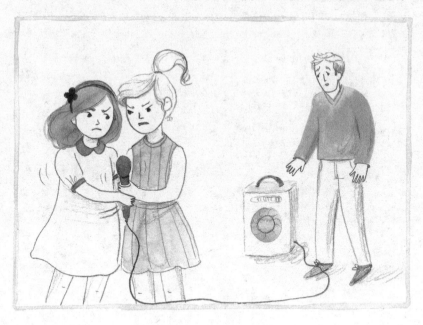

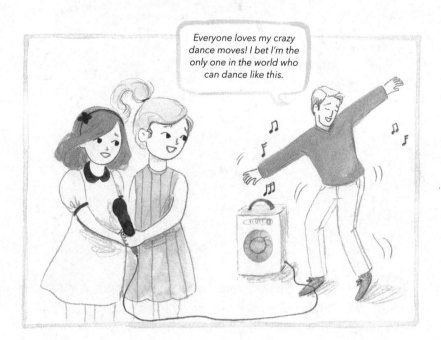

HELP YOUR CHILD PIVOT PLAYFULLY AWAY FROM CONFLICT.

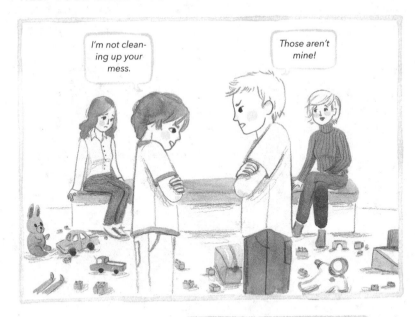

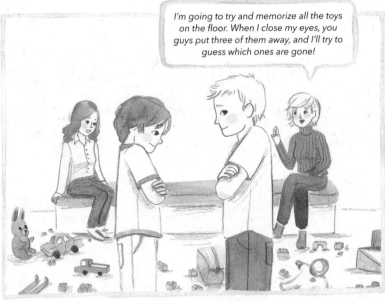

Injecting playful invitations into a difficult parenting situation can not only calm things down; it can often shift things to get kids to work together, giving them practice at having positive and cooperative interactions, which can be built on for the future. While this may be temporarily distracting them from the conflict, that isn't the goal. Rather, the aim is to shift the interaction to a more productive one. When your kids get repeated experiences joining together with you, coupled with really positive emotion and fun, you're helping them set that relational tone. What's fun, enjoyable, and pleasant we want more of. If you want your kids to enjoy their siblings and friends and put in more effort to make the relationship work, play is a good way to begin to facilitate that.

It's like flipping a switch that lights up the playful brain! Whatever conflict or negative pattern you were about to see gives way to joining together. You're left with a child who is much more willing, even eager, to join in, take things in a positive direction, solve problems, and elevate mundane tasks with creativity and laughter. And kids learn the implicit message that life, and even tricky situations, can become fun, even when we have to do things we don't like, because a loving parent has modeled and engaged with the kids in play's ability to transform the moment.

Playful Pitfalls to Avoid

A few warnings about shifting misbehavior with the playful pivot: First, don't attempt to turn every behavioral issue into a race or competition (like a contest between siblings to see who can get all their toys cleaned up first). That can work if kids are still fairly regulated, but if their bodies are tense and they're talking to you through gritted teeth, that might not be the best time to pivot playfully. There's a chance that the strategy will work, but you'll need to really tune in to your child before you proceed.

Likewise, don't attempt to turn every negative emotion or challenge into a big-energy play moment. Sometimes your child might need a quieter, slower moment of connection. In this case, try getting down to your child's level and pulling them close, attuning to what they're feeling, and offering help or asking them what they might need. We don't want to just rev things into turbo-fun mode as the answer to every bump in the road or negative emotion. Parents also need to create and honor the space and time for their child to feel difficult emotions, where they're not distracted from feelings, pressured to mask what they're experiencing, or having to be light and fun when that isn't where they are. It can be a huge miss if we're being silly and fun and cheerleading when our child needs to cry and be held. Our goal is *not* to use play to keep our kids from feeling but rather to use playfulness in an attuned way to relate and create positive connection.

> Parents also need to create and honor the space and time for their child to feel difficult emotions, where they're not distracted from feelings, pressured to mask what they're experiencing, or having to be light and fun when that isn't where they are. It can be a huge miss if we're being silly and fun when our child needs to cry and be held.

What's more, getting kids to burst into the giggles is awesome, but this isn't about teasing, doing a comedy routine, or getting big belly laughs. Your child might actually feel worse if the joke's on them, leaving them further dysregulated. Again, you want to know your child and tune in to what they're feeling as well as possible.

Don't be afraid to try new things as you play. Novelty isn't just good—it's often totally necessary. If your child thinks a particular pivot is always funny, then great; they might laugh and put their shoes on every time you pretend to painfully squeeze your feet into their tiny sandals. In that case you've likely created a beautifully memorable routine.

But if an old pivot is getting stale, don't be afraid to come up with something new and ignite more creativity. Maybe next time, you accidentally put their teeny shoes on your ears and ask if they like your earrings! Either way, you're helping them associate putting on their shoes with novelty and fun—key ingredients not only for gaining cooperation but also for building a flexible brain.

All that said, the point isn't really to distract your kids from having to deal with situations that can build resilience and relational skills. As we've said, sometimes you're going to simply allow them to sit with the disappointment or frustration of not getting their way. They have to learn about getting along in the world, after all, and the way they become resilient is by practicing walking through challenging moments and emotions, with enough support and care from us.

But if you can add fun and laughter to challenging moments that threaten to spiral out of control, you can often lighten the mood and bring your kids back to regulation enough that you can *then* teach the lessons you want to share, once the emotional storm has passed. Sometimes that might mean addressing the earlier situation.

AFTER THINGS HAVE CALMED DOWN,
YOU CAN ADDRESS THE EARLIER CONFLICT.

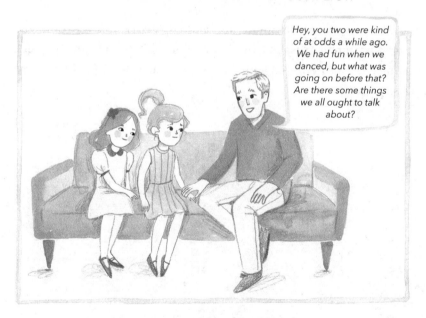

Hey, you two were kind of at odds a while ago. We had fun when we danced, but what was going on before that? Are there some things we all ought to talk about?

At other times, you can highlight the positive emotions the two of you just shared.

Again, you don't throw out the rules, and *of course* you want to continue teaching your kids the lessons they need to learn. But if you

AFTER THINGS HAVE CALMED DOWN,
HIGHLIGHT THE POSITIVES.

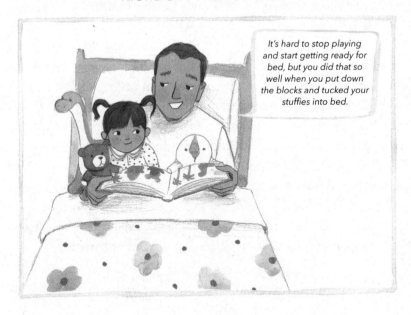

can use play to defuse the tension and negativity in a situation, and send the signals of safety that play often does, you'll find it much simpler to both enforce your limits and teach the points you want them to learn.

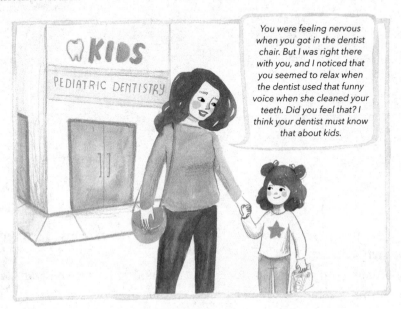

The Playful Point

Ultimately, the point is that we can use playfulness not just during set-aside playtimes but all throughout the day. In fact, everything we've discussed throughout the book has been focused less on specific strategies or approaches and more on an overall mindset, *a way of being with our kids.*

Play matters. And what you do with your kids matters. When you spend time with them each day enjoying each other, laughing and joining, even in small doses, you take steps toward helping them develop into secure, confident, strong-minded individuals who feel cared for and who know how to love. They'll grow up with a greater potential to combat stress, perform under pressure, and address problems with a spirit of competence, courage, and fun that will serve them well.

If our children can learn from a tender age that they are surrounded by available sources of comfort, care, and encouragement, they will be more likely to have a healthy nervous system, regulated body rhythms, and a balanced and receptive mind—all working together in beautiful harmony. These are the skills you're building as you play with your kids, and as you allow play to pervade the various aspects of your relationship. This is why we called this book *The Way of Play.* Play isn't just something we *do* to pass the time. It's a *way of being* as a parent. Play is kids' primary language, and it's key to helping them build emotional, cognitive, and relational skills. And most importantly, it's a way you can build a stronger relationship with them that will reward you both for years to come.

Acknowledgments

From Tina and Georgie

What a privilege it has been to work with our wonderful editor, Marnie Cochran, who has been wise, encouraging, and insightful from start to finish. Thank you for giving us exactly the input and support we needed at every step, Marnie, as we teamed up to make the way of play more possible, practical, and purposeful for future generations.

We'd like to thank our literary agents, Doug Abrams and Rachel Neumann, for their passion and care as we brought these ideas from imagination to reality. Thank you, Rachel, for helping us run with a creative spark and for sharing our belief that play is important and healthy at every stage of parenting. And Doug, we will always be deeply grateful to have you as a trusted advisor, dear friend, and steadfast supporter of the mission to bring greater well-being, stronger connection, and more joy into the lives of parents and children. Thanks to Sarah Rainone for your help in the final stretch.

We greatly appreciate the artistic talent of Merrilee Liddiard, an illustrator who brought so much depth of meaning to the drawings that accompany each of the PlayStrong concepts. Merrilee, we thank you for mirroring our ideas and bringing little moments to life by illustrating play so intuitively, effectively, and beautifully. In doing so, you've made childhood appear even more magical.

Much appreciation to Rebecca Knowles, Jamie Chaves, Olivia Martinez-Hauge, and Amanda Staples, who provided very helpful feedback on sensory integration and processing from their skilled lenses as occupational therapists. And thank you to the other invaluable readers and friends who gave feedback on the book or design elements: Dan Siegel, Brett Kirby, Elizabeth Olson, Jennifer Shim Lovers, Stacy Dever Levy, Michael Thompson, and Adrienne Hollingsworth.

To our team at The Center for Connection, it's such an honor to do this important work with you as we collectively nurture kids, families, and other individuals so they can be happy, healthy, balanced, and resilient. So many of you shared your expertise in ways that have influenced the concepts we teach that it would be impossible to thank you all individually, but we appreciate each one of you as professionals committed to affirming and working from our shared lens and whole-brain perspective.

And to our colleagues from the Play Strong Institute, we are thankful for your generosity, service, and collaboration as we support children with the power of play. We want to extend our deepest appreciation to our remarkable play therapy faculty: Jennifer Shim Lovers, Annalise Kordell, Felisha Cullum, Rebekah Springs, and Sharon Tan. To those who have trained with us, thank you for sharing the therapeutic benefits of play and our unique approach with kids and their caregivers all over the world. We gratefully acknowledge Sharon Berg and Judi Stadler at Para Los Niños, Kelli Carroll and Denise Matsuyama at UCLA Mattel Children's Hospital, Louise Godbold and Lindsay Evangelista at ECHO Training, Lisa Clements and Kristen Metzger at Kidspace Children's Museum, and Thayer Case and Emma Pile at Maverick Psychotherapy, for our enjoyable and productive training partnerships. Thank you for being champions for PlayStrong and spreading its potential to the families you reach!

And finally, we extend our humble gratitude to all the families who have touched our lives by working with us in some capacity over the years. Maybe at some point you've known us in our clinical practices or attended one of Tina's educational workshops or gotten down on the floor with your kid (or been a kid!) in Georgie's playroom. What an honor for us to witness your growth, to see your love and dedication, and to help your children develop into mature, self-aware individuals full of empathy and hope. We haven't revealed your names or details in the writing of this book, but a composite of your experiences of parenting and playing with your kids has informed our thinking and helped us hone the PlayStrong strategies for more effective teaching. Thus we gather this collective wisdom—your wisdom included—to offer even more families new skills and examples that may revive play as a powerful pathway to understand and communicate with our children, reduce conflict, take care of their emotions and behavior, build positive memories, and create loving relationships to last a lifetime. When they look back, we know your kids will always remember the way you played.

From Georgie

To Tina, you inspire me with your great wisdom, passion for teaching, and never-ending energy to deepen connections. I have enjoyed every moment we've spent dreaming big and bringing the message of play to the world. The collaboration with you and Scott, who guided the many drafts of this book with his own literary talent, editorial input, and parenting knowledge, has been an absolute gift. I will carry it deep in my heart. With your unwavering trust, empathy, and optimism, the two of you have influenced the parent, professional, and person I am in countless ways.

To Jack, my best teacher in play, you bring such light to the world simply by being yourself. Your open mind and heart, caring spirit, sense of humor, insightful and inventive brain, and passion for nature are part of the magic of who you are. In your unique growth, you have taught me to attune and connect with the way *you* play, and you show me how to love you more deeply and authentically every single day. Your dad and I thank our lucky stars that we get to be your parents. We delight in you!

To Justin, thank you for being a partner in life who lives for the thrill of new ideas and ventures. If anyone knows how to make work feel more like play, it is you. You've shown that a family can thrive by staying true to a vision, and it has been such a fun and meaningful journey to raise Jack with you. Thank you for your unconditional support of my professional work and the writing of this book. This is *our* achievement—I'm thrilled I get to share this joy with you.

I want to thank the extraordinary teachers and mentors who have played a pivotal role in my development, offering their fierce intelligence, passion for helping families, and genuine care for me: Alison Green, Ann-Marie John, Christine Campbell, Amy Johnson, Susan Spitzer, Mona Delahooke, Fan Zhang, and Ben Grey. With great affection I recognize my close collaborator, Rebecca Bokoch, for your infinite patience as you share your gift for research with me. A special mention to Stacy Dever Levy, Ashlee Bixby, Crystal Ross, Priya Agarwal, Catherine Kelly, Amber Hughes, Raji Natrajan-Tyagi, Justine Plocher, Sandi Sickels, ZhiZhen Tao, Claire Rokey, Ledette Gambini, Robyn Park, Adrienne Hollingsworth, Carly Nalbandian, Dahlia Bagnis, and Olivia Martinez-Hauge, who make me proud to be a fellow play practitioner.

To our dearest friends who are the most loving and playful people to their children, we are profoundly blessed to call you family: Sarah Pyle, Shane Lynch, and Jude; Brett and Natalia Kennedy, Naia and Alyra. To Juli Agajanian, my best friend of thirty years, having so many memories with you is worth more than gold.

To my parents, Marty and Jody Wisen, you've taught me to dig deep and build tenacity and resilience. I want to thank my mother-in-law, Florence Vincent, who was the first to encourage me to write a book. To my aunt Leslie Wilson, thank you for cheering me on. To my sister-in-law, Sarah Jane Vincent, you inspire me as a strong woman entrepreneur. Justin and I are incredibly proud of you. To my sister, Carrie Wisen, you are the most gifted early childhood educator

I've ever seen, and your deep understanding of young children has influenced me in profound ways. I marvel as you raise your daughters, Linley and Marin, with such warmth, insight, and empathy. And to my grandparents Lelah and Herb Wilson, a couple of characters who made me laugh and nurtured the PlayStrong spirit in me; I celebrate your memory in every page of this book.

From Tina

What a gift you are, Georgie! You bring incredible wisdom and passion for the art and science of play therapy, but you also have the gift of teaching parents and clinicians the transformational possibilities of the power of play. You embody the joyfulness and endless creativity of imagination that come with play, and I'm so glad we're getting to share that together with our readers.

To my love, Scott, thank you for all that you do to make this work happen. It truly wouldn't be birthed into the world without your dedication, generosity, and especially your editorial and writing talents. I love the life we've built. And I look forward to many years of play ahead.

To my parents—Deborah Buckwalter (the world's best human and mother), Galen Buckwalter, Judy and Bill Ramsey, and Jay Bryson— thank you for always loving us and our boys fiercely.

Ben, Luke, and JP, I adore you. You have taught me so much, and while I got really bored of banging "superguys" into one another from time to time, playing with you three when you were little was such a gift. Filling your pockets, putting tools or sharp things you found in your homemade belts, creating worlds, breaking windows, designing magic shows, building forts, "wrestling," and a million more forgotten moments brought me so much joy. JP, your contagious full-body laughter that makes you out of breath; Luke, your unique way of seeing the world (and sometimes unknown worlds); and Ben, your delight from hitting my bad pitches over and over in the backyard, and your intense love of playing with us—your minds, your hearts, and your imaginations took my breath away. Play looks different now that you're older, but when we hang out, it's still my favorite thing in the universe.

A huge shout-out to my favorite playmates in my later grown-up years. First, my friends who make me laugh the most and with whom I enjoy the *best* playdates, the HBOS: Lynn Hayes, Jordan Hayes, Liz Olson, Steve Olson, Sonia Singla, and Neil Singla. Scott and I couldn't be luckier. I adore you all. And to my newer friends, Aliza Pressman and Dana Klein, I look forward to many years ahead of gut-wrenching laughter at ourselves.

I want to share my deep-felt gratitude for my colleague and dear friend, Dan Siegel. My years learning from you, creating and sharing our work together, and our continued friendship are incredible gifts that I hold dearly. Thank you to my other colleagues, teachers, and friends who ground me, encourage me, challenge me, and join with me to make an impact in the world: Mona Delahooke; (the "other") Michael Thompson; Susan Stiffelman; Janet Lansbury; Cara Natterson; Vanessa Kroll Bennett; my "author squad" made up of Catherine-Reynolds Lewis, Debbie Reber, Julie Lythcott-Haims, Ned Johnson, Katie Hurley, Jessica Lahey, Catherine Steiner-Adair, Michele Borba, Madeline Levine, Devorah Heitner, Nefertiti Austin, Phyllis Fagell, Audrey Monke, and Christine Koh. And thank you to my team at The Center for Connection for all you teach me and how you change lives every day. I want to give a special shout-out to our incredible leadership team—Hanna Novak, Cathy Schaefer, Olivia Martinez-Hauge, Will Lacey, Tami Millard, Orli Lahav, Desiree Misrachi, Annalise Kordell, Jennifer Shim Lovers, Deborah Buckwalter, and Maura Cook.

And a special shout-out to my incredible work partner of many years, Ayla Dillard. Really, there aren't enough words to express what a gift you are to me, and everyone you interact with. You bring light, and love, and brilliance, and kindness, and creativity, and talent, and equanimity to every micro-moment, and I don't know what I would do without you. You embody everything I teach and strive for, and you are a *huge* part of the impact that my work makes in the world. You make everything happen so that I can be present in my work and in my time with my family and friends, and you make sure to remind me to play and care for myself, too. You're truly the best, and I'm so grateful for you and your gifts. Thank you for all you are and all you do.

The Practicalities of Creating a Play Space for Your Child—and for You

Many of us hold the idea that kids can play at the drop of a hat—anywhere, anytime. Sometimes that's the case, but when possible, we want to create an environment that encourages their highest forms of creativity, focus, and self-direction. The best play spaces grow with your child: from a baby rolling on a mat grasping at cups and rings, to toddlers climbing and exploring, on up to older kids designing their own games, tinkering, and pretending. Here we want to help you think about how to set up an environment that's just what your child needs.

First, how does your child usually play at this age, and what kind of play atmosphere do you want to cultivate in your home? Would you and your child rather play tucked away in a quiet corner? Or freely roam around, allowing for more sound, movement, and variety? Most likely, there will be times when one or the other approach is preferred.

Sometimes you two might prefer a designated hub where toys are kept and play-builds can happen, such as your child's bedroom or a playroom. Or you might want to create a system for using and tidying toys around the entire living area. In other words, we might be talking about one part of one room, one room, or the entire place where you live. Every family has their own culture at home; just go with what works best for you, your space, and your way of play.

Whatever space you establish as the play hub, there are some specifics that can help you make that area incredible for your child. It all comes down to *setting*, *sight*, and *stuff*.

SETTING

A thoughtfully designed play space should be equally appealing to you and your child. If you can create a space where the whole family feels comfortable, then you're all more likely to spend time being together there, enjoying one another as you play.

It doesn't have to be fully designed or cost a lot of money—not at all. What's much more important is that it's comfortable. Maybe you find a second-hand chair you love to curl up in and read together, or a cushion with the perfect degree of softness for sitting on the floor. Maybe the colors or artwork on the walls just feel cozy and inviting to you.

A tiny kid-sized table with chairs is good. But what's even better, if you have the space, is to get a sturdy, oversized coffee table with room enough for several of you to gather around for art projects, games, and puzzles. If you can get one second-hand, even better—because it'll likely get scuffed or marked up with paint or pens. If you want, you can add casters so the table moves out of the way when your child needs more space for play on the floor. A neutral area rug is a visual canvas for kids to dive into serious floor play and construction.

Keep in mind, too, when you think about setting, that there's almost nothing better than playing outside. Spending time outdoors might be even more crucial than setting up a playroom in your home. There are literally *hundreds* of studies proclaiming the benefits of playing in nature—it's good for your child's immune system, physical strength, mental health, and more. That applies whether kids are digging in the dirt, planting a garden, collecting fallen leaves and sticks, going on walks or hikes, climbing trees, swinging, stargazing, or playing in water—all of these activities are therapeutic and important for kids.

You can approach being outdoors like a child's playground, without boundaries. Or you can create a hub for play outside if you have the space. If you have a yard, set up a kid-sized table, along with seating and a small storage shelf, and maybe a play kitchen. Think of this hub as a makerspace where your kids can bring their toys or create with natural objects like leaves, twigs, and pebbles. A bench, picnic table, or blanket on the grass can serve the same purpose if you go to the park.

SIGHT

One important factor that you might not think about is sight, or what your kids see in the play place you're creating. Toys that are out of sight are out of mind. But when play materials can be seen, a child's imagination fires up.

Sure, you might love the idea of neatly organized baskets on shelves, with the toys tidily tucked away. But set up your playroom that way and you're likely to be met with shrugged shoulders and the statement, "There's nothing to do." If toys are buried in baskets or hidden, they often don't exist in the child's mind's eye.

Does that mean toys need to be sprawled all across the room? Not at all. Feel free to use those baskets and bins. But save them for larger or odd-shaped objects and display them on the floor so kids can see what's inside them. Maybe throw a bunch of the same type of toy in a bin—possibly all the toy cars or a bunch of action figures.

What gets displayed on shelves, if you have them, could be a small but organized collection of different types of toys, each with its own prized position. If you really need to put smaller toys in containers on a shelf, try to keep them organized by type in see-through bins or containers that have a low side so kids can see into them.

Pro tip: Rotate your collections of toys. Instead of leaving everything on display at all times, keep most of your toys in storage. In other words, have a limited set of toys out for open play, displayed at or below a child's eye level and within reach, but keep plenty of toys out of sight in what some families call the "toy library" (aka closet, attic, or basement). Rotating "new" toys into the play space can keep it fresh and interesting. Children often rediscover old toys that have been in the "library" for a while as if new all over again. If you aren't sure how many toys to put out at once, think of Georgie's Ten-Minute Rule: If you need more than ten minutes to clean up everything, there are too many toys on display.

In short, the more visible the materials, the more creative the play.

STUFF

Not all toys are created equal. Indeed, the kinds of toys you offer your child can make a difference to the whole organization of their play. So how do you know which toys to make available?

We recommend offering a balance of some of the cool toys on the market—you know, the kind grandparents love to send at the holidays—and classic, open-ended toys, like action figures, dolls, blocks, cars, and balls, all of which can be used in a multitude of ways as your child grows and develops into new stages of play and learning.

Here's a brief list of classic toy categories aligned with the PlayStrong philosophy to deepen and diversify your child's play (roughly ages two to ten). Keep in mind that there's no definitive or right set of toys kids need. But these examples—some for indoors, some for outdoors—can give you an idea of how you can provide a good variety of options for play. You don't have to own all of these toys, by the way. Many of them can be found in a neighborhood playground or play space in your community, and going to them (instead of having them at home) is almost always a good idea, since that'll give your kids a variety of play-based experiences.

Sensory toys: Promote brain-body balance and regulation
- Play dough
- Sand and sand toys (bucket, shovel, rake)

- Natural objects (shells, twigs, leaves, etc.)
- Recyclable items (containers, cardboard, etc.)
- Fidget toys
- Play silks or fabrics
- Pillows and blankets

Full-body toys: Expand gross motor skills and impulse control
- Swing
- Balance board
- Climbing rope
- Slide
- Cushions or beanbag chair
- Tent (can be homemade from a sheet over a table)

Creative toys: Build fine motor skills, self-expression, and confidence
- Drawing utensils (crayons, markers, pencils, etc.)
- Paints and paintbrushes
- Glue, tape, scissors
- Paper
- Crafting materials
- Chalkboard and chalk
- Musical instruments (drum, xylophone, pots and pans with wooden spoons, etc.)
- Children's books

Construction toys and games: Develop visual, spatial, and executive skills and flexibility
- Legos
- Building blocks
- Magnet tiles
- Construction tool set
- Cars, trucks, planes, boats
- Puzzles
- Board games

Expressive toys: Engage, express, and manage emotions
- Puppets
- Stuffed wild animals
- Dinosaurs
- Action figures (heroes and villains)
- Foam swords
- Soft foam balls

Nurturing toys: Teach empathy and caring behavior
- Farm set and animals
- Stuffed domestic animals (dogs, cats, birds, etc.)
- Baby doll, bottle, clothes, care items
- Play tea set
- Play kitchen
- Play food and dishes

Dramatic play toys: Experience storytelling and understanding of real-world interactions
- Costumes and hats
- Dollhouse, furniture, and family
- Play medical kit (stethoscope, bandages, etc.)
- Telephones or walkie-talkies
- Cash register and play money
- Treasure chest

We recommend collecting a selection of items from each category to provide your child with a wide array of experiences, from nurturing toys to the kind that let kids feel fierce, along with constructive and dramatic play options.

Just be sure play items are appropriate for your child's unique developmental stage by checking age ranges marked on toys and games. After all, toddlers typically benefit from a different set of sensorimotor objects and educational toys than school-aged kids. Each needs age-appropriate toys and games to scaffold their developing skills. If your child with individual differences is developing play on their own timetable, then meeting their unique preferences and sensory needs in your choice of toys is much more important than the age marked on the box.

And don't forget to include common household items as "toys." Objects like coffee canisters, bowls, wooden spoons, yarn, cardboard boxes, and masking tape are prime examples of open-ended objects that kids can use in a million different ways. As a child who adored making pillow forts and sock puppets once said, "My favorite toys aren't toys. They are anything where I can make something out of nothing."

Setting, sight, and stuff. Stay focused on these factors and you'll set up a play area you and your kids will love. You don't need a fancy playroom with expensive toys and all the trimmings. And there's no official rule saying you must use all-natural, sustainable wooden toys with organic paint and biodegradable finish imported from Europe that cost hundreds of dollars and make your whole house look like a Waldorf or Montessori classroom.

Just use your knowledge of your child, follow their lead, and set things up the way that makes the most sense to you. Then have a ball playing with your kid.

Designing a Play-Based World for Our Children (and Ourselves)

It's imperative that our culture recognize the value of play and work toward creating environments where children can thrive relationally, mentally, and emotionally. We therefore encourage those who care about the mental health and well-being of children to adopt the following provisions to protect and promote children's right to healthy forms of play.

INFANTS

Play represents a baby's first drive to learn and acquire important sensory, motor, cognitive, and emotional skills. Infants need to engage with sensitive and attuned caregivers in free exploration and play at regular intervals throughout the day. The American Academy of Pediatrics has even urged doctors to provide "prescriptions for play" at well-baby checks.

Even in the case of newborns, a parent or caregiver's access to adequate childcare, social-parenting education, support networks, and safe places to play with their children impacts healthy developmental and parent-child interactions.

TODDLERS AND PRESCHOOLERS

Optimal toddler and preschool systems of learning emphasize models in which the teacher engages students in activities within a child's zone of proximal development. Early learning and brain development are ideally supported by a child's intrinsic drive to develop skills through joyful exploration, unencumbered by external demands such as drills and rote activities. We therefore strongly encourage a preschool curriculum primarily based on skill building through engagement in free play. Preschools and daycares (serving infants to age four) should thus offer primarily play-based emergent curricula to honor the early brain development of each child and their specific developmental play needs.

PRE-K KIDS

As policymakers create opportunities for more enrollment in pre-kindergarten programs, there is some debate about introducing didactic teaching earlier compared to less-structured play models. It remains important for four- and five-year-olds in pre-K environments to be allowed to play for the majority of the day. "Sit still, eyes on me" can have an adverse impact on behavior and on later school learning if introduced too soon. We highly recommend taking preventative steps in pre-K to enhance future school success by providing nurturing relationships with teachers and letting children build more mature cognitive skills through free and guided play.

KINDERGARTNERS

The increased push for table-top and full-day academic learning in kindergarten, which used to be devoted mostly to free play, has created more anxiety for many children at the start of elementary school. Younger learners need additional time to develop key abilities in paying attention, managing impulses, and planning their actions before they should be expected to sit for long periods and produce test scores. Kindergartners need plenty of playtime to scaffold the fundamental motor, language, executive functioning, and emotional regulation skills needed to be successful once they are ready for structured learning. Homework is not needed at this age; children should be playing after school for several hours per day.

ELEMENTARY STUDENTS

First through fifth and sixth graders should be given plenty of recess time, more access to performing and expressive arts, and frequent movement breaks, preferably outdoors as much as possible. Doing so can increase learning, ease transitions, and help focus. Shortening recess to, for example, twenty minutes does not offer students enough time to fully organize their play and receive its benefits.

We especially discourage taking away recess as a behavioral measure, as it can produce detrimental effects on a student's physical and mental health, not to mention their overall conduct. At least one full hour of recess per day would be considered the minimum amount of free play needed for elementary students while at school. Elementary schools that have prioritized recess have observed students' improved relationships with peers and adults and increased the educational value of this unstructured time.

Recess options besides sports gear and playground equipment should be available in order to promote a wider repertoire of play beyond competitive games. Other materials can include those that foster pretend and dramatic play (like costumes); music, dance, and movement (like instruments); art and creativity (like paint and chalk); and nature-based activities (like shovels, pails, seeds, etc.). A decreased amount of homework at this age will allow for more hours of healthy, unstructured play after school.

MIDDLE AND HIGH SCHOOL STUDENTS

Older kids should have opportunities for outdoor education and access to green spaces as well—not just taking the occasional lesson outside but incorporating more hands-on, real-world skills and experiential study for extended periods of playful outdoor learning. Upper schools we've worked with who regularly devote time for mindfulness and meditative practices, art and movement activities, and regular nature-based field trips have noticed improvements in student functioning.

Adult-led physical education and organized athletics can help teens stay active, but these structured (and often performance-based) activities should not substitute for the freedom of outdoor enrichment. Adolescence is a critical period for supporting students' emotional health. Screen-free activities that help young people feel connected with creativity, the natural world, community, and their cultural identities also decrease feelings of isolation and augment secure, stable, and nurturing relationships that buffer against toxic levels of stress and build emotional resilience.

ADULTS

It's not just our kids who benefit from play. By continuing to play into our adult years, we can further integrate many parts of the brain that help us think, focus, remember, and feel more energized. Our play looks different from when we were kids, of course. You might even be thinking that you can't even imagine what play would look like in adulthood. Remember, play is doing something just because it's fun, just for the pleasure of it! So finding activities we enjoy doing for ourselves now that we have grown-up interests can provide us with the kinds of social connection, stress relief, delight, and emotional regulation that, in turn, enable us to become more invigorated and present as parents. Infusing more playfulness and joy into our adult personalities, and even our work, can create lasting change in our approach to life, health, family, learning, and even work.

So go ahead: Sign up for that dance class or pickleball lesson, or set up a coffee with that friend who makes you laugh. We know it's hard to find time for fun when the kids demand *so many* of our resources—and we don't want to add self-care to the list of obligations you already feel. But see if you can find just a few ways to play and enjoy little moments on a regular basis. When you do, you'll be taking better care of yourself, you'll be modeling playfulness across the lifespan, and you'll have more to offer your children as well.

The Way of Play

By Tina Payne Bryson and Georgie Wisen-Vincent

By spending just a few minutes each day playing with your child, you can not only enjoy a stronger relationship with them but also better understand them, build and strengthen their cognitive and relational skills, and reduce the amount of time you spend disciplining and addressing misbehavior. Here are the various PlayStrong strategies we discuss in the book.

PLAYSTRONG STRATEGY #1:
Think Out Loud

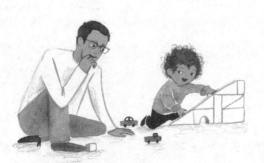

Notice, as you and your child play, what you see them doing. Name what you see, especially with an eye toward describing their mind and intentions. Doing so will deepen the relationship between you and plant the seed that it's possible to pay attention to one's own thoughts as well as those of another.

Primary skill being developed in the child: Awareness of their inner world: thoughts, feelings, wishes, intentions, and more.

Primary message received by the child: Someone understands me, and I can understand myself.

Make Yourself a Mirror

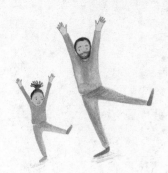

Watch for ways to use your body, face, and voice (your BFVs) to mirror your child's simple but important signals. Simply reflect back what you see. Doing so will allow them to recognize how people bond, and it will help them tap into emotional connection and build empathy.

Primary skill being developed in the child: A deeper understanding of their own emotional life, which can deepen connection with and empathy for others.

Primary message received by the child: Someone tunes in to me. I can tune in to others.

Bring Emotions to Life

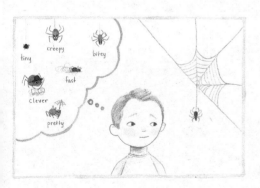

Introduce the language of feelings into playtime, thus strengthening the emotionally intelligent, meaning-making connections between your child's body and brain.

Primary skill being developed in the child: The ability to recognize, manage, and express emotions.

Primary message received by the child: Someone will help me recognize and make sense of my big feelings.

Dial Intensity Up or Down

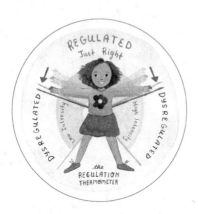

When you see your child getting out of control or having big emotional responses during play, first chase the why. Be curious about where the reactions are coming from. Then, look for ways to bring calmness or energy, depending on the situation and what you know of your child.

Primary skill being developed in the child: An ability to regulate their emotions and actions when they're upset and struggling.

Primary message received by the child: Someone is going to be here for me when I'm out of control and can't handle things very well by myself.

Scaffold and Stretch

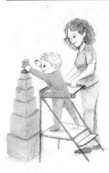

Provide supportive scaffolding opportunities that can stretch your child to grow. Offer encouragement and step in when necessary. But let them struggle when appropriate so they can broaden their skills and allow their emotional regulation and executive function to work together.

Primary skill being developed in the child: Resilience in the face of difficult situations.

Primary message received by the child: Someone is going to show up for me when things get hard, and I can handle more than I think I can.

Narrate to Integrate

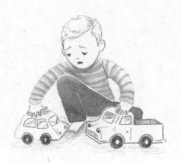

Tune in to the stories that emerge during playtime, using them to build skills around handling fears, dealing with conflict, and understanding the self. Allow the storytelling to remain fun—that's crucial—but watch for ways to elevate the narrative into something more meaningful.

Primary skill being developed in the child: Use of stories to better comprehend and deal with difficult circumstances.

Primary message received by the child: I can use stories to better understand what's going on around me, then make choices that are good for me and that help me take charge of a situation.

Set Playtime Parameters

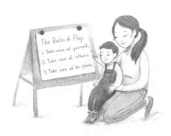

Let your child lead, but playtime shouldn't become a free-for-all. By setting appropriate and well-defined boundaries that clearly communicate your expectations, you give your child opportunities to develop new skills they can use to respect the rules of a situation and act in ways that benefit them and the world around them.

Primary skill being developed in the child: Flexibility and adaptability to help them work within boundaries and make positive decisions.

Primary message received by the child: Someone is going to keep me safe and help me learn to do that for myself.

Index

About the Authors

TINA PAYNE BRYSON, PHD, LCSW, is the co-author (with Daniel J. Siegel) of two *New York Times* bestsellers—*The Whole-Brain Child* and *No-Drama Discipline*—each of which has been translated into over fifty languages, with *The Whole-Brain Child* selling more than a million copies. She is also the author of *The Bottom Line for Baby* and co-author (with Daniel J. Siegel) of *The Power of Showing Up* and *The Yes Brain*. Bryson is a psychotherapist, as well as a founder and the executive director of The Center for Connection, multidisciplinary clinical practices in Pasadena and Santa Barbara, California; the Play Strong Institute, a center devoted to the study, research, and practice of play therapy through a neurodevelopment lens; and The Center for Connection and Neurodiversity, a wing of The Center for Connection devoted to celebrating neurodifferences and providing brain-based occupational therapy across the lifespan.

Bryson keynotes conferences and conducts workshops for parents, educators, clinicians, and industry leaders all over the world. She consults with various companies and organizations, including the Texas Education Agency, along with the Nike Sport Research Lab, where she was project director for mental or emotional performance for the Dreamweaver Program. She is a graduate of Baylor University and earned her doctorate from the University of Southern California, where her research explored attachment science, child development, and the field of interpersonal neurobiology. Tina Payne Bryson lives in Los Angeles with her husband and their three children.

TinaBryson.com
Facebook.com/TinaPayneBrysonPhd
Instagram: @TinaPayneBryson
X: @TinaBryson
TheCenterforConnection.org

GEORGIE WISEN-VINCENT, LMFT, RPT-S, is a nationally recognized play therapy expert and the co-founder, with Tina Payne Bryson, of the Play Strong Institute. A graduate professor and active researcher in childhood play, attachment science, and mental health, Wisen-Vincent has been commissioned as a consultant, program designer, and lead trainer for several major organizations and frequently presents to educators, parents, and clinical professionals on the power of play-driven learning. She completed advanced study in play therapy at the University of Roehampton, London, and gained specialist endorsement in early childhood mental health. Georgie Wisen-Vincent is a child, adolescent, and family psychotherapist in private practice in Los Angeles.

GeorgieVincent.com
Facebook.com/GeorgieWisenVincent
Instagram: @georgiewisenvincent
X: @georgiewvincent

About the Type

This book was set in Minion, a 1990 Adobe Originals typeface by Robert Slimbach. Minion is inspired by classical, old-style typefaces of the late Renaissance, a period of elegant and beautiful type designs. Created primarily for text setting, Minion combines the aesthetic and functional qualities that make text type highly readable with the versatility of digital technology.